THRIVE

A mom's guide to staying sane and healthy amidst the chaos of modern family life

Dina Vecchione Milne

Thrive

ISBN: 978-1-7350668-0-6

Thrive

DEDICATION

For my dad who taught me the three most important lessons in life. First, stand up for what you believe in, even if it means getting your ass kicked. Second, don't be a follower …you never know where you'll end up. Third, keep a straight face so you don't give away your hand and never hit on a 13 when the dealer has a 6 showing.

CONTENTS

ACKNOWLEDGMENTS

While I bring this book to you as a Health Coach, I also bring a background in social work, which has provided me with vital information and experience relevant to the writing of this book. Throughout my career as a social worker, I have had the privilege of working with countless mothers and families, many of whom struggled with the same issues that I address in this book. I learned so much from each and every one of them and I thank them for allowing me this first-hand look into their lives. That being said, the most important role I have ever had, the one that gives me the most experience and valuable insight is that of being a mom. Before my children, I could never have imagined the incredible joys or the great challenges of being a mother. Each of my amazing children has brought something unique and wonderful to my life and I learn from them every day. To each of them, I say thank you for being you and for opening your minds to new possibilities. The world is yours, find your Dharma!

~Mimibewhasu

PREFACE

When I first began writing this book I designed it to be a quick read. The reason for this is that I am well aware that my audience does not have time to leisurely sit and read. They are moms like me and busy doesn't begin to scratch the surface. So, for me anything that I wanted to read came in the car with me. This way I could read it piece meal while waiting for my kids to come out of school, picking up from practice, etc. This was literally my only down time, if you could call that downtime.

As I was sure that there were other moms out there facing many of the same challenges I have faced, this book is written for them. It is an account of my own journey to improve my physical and mental health, which I think many of you will relate to. This book also contains clear, concise tips and practical advice for those of you who are still struggling.

As modern moms we are on the clock 24/7, whether that be at work, working at home, taking care of family, acting as a taxi driver, running errands or taking care of other obligations. We have been somewhat programmed to believe that if we do anything less than everything then we have failed. In this book I will explore the various reasons that so-called logic is faulty. As a matter of fact, this logic can best be described as complete and total bull. We will look at these beliefs as well as how individually and collectively we can change them.

Keep this book in on your car to read while you are waiting for your kids or wherever you can steal a few minutes for yourself. Even if you only read a page or two a week, I promise you will be happy that you did.

There are a few words that you will hear frequently throughout this book. The words are liberating, empowering and free. The reason for this is that this book is written to help you set yourself free from those things that are impeding your progress toward physical and emotional wellness. I wish you all the best on your journey.

Now let's get started.

Inspiration

One day while watching my daughter's hockey game I realized that my story was not mine alone. I was sitting with a bunch of other moms when one started talking about how stressed out, she was. The fact is, she was saying out loud what many of us felt. She said that between work and kids, cleaning and getting everyone where they need to be, she didn't know which end was up. As the mother of four, there was a constant request for her attention, which she said she wants to give but is just being pulled in too many directions. Wherever she is, she is thinking about other obligations and how she is going to get everything done. There was always someone or something pulling at her. At times she admitted feeling like she can hardly breathe.

As someone who appears on the outside to really have her shit together, I was shocked to hear this, but it made me realize something. Appearances are just that. I thought to myself... if she is struggling, how many others are struggling? Well, I got a snippet of this answer as she had barely finished venting when five other moms (me being one of them) jumped right in with similar stories. All of us stressed, all of us experiencing some type of inflammation and fatigue, and all of us feeling like our juggling acts were failing. What did this tell me? Out of nine people sitting on this little section of bleachers that day, six of us were experiencing the same type of stress. I should note that the other three people on the bleachers consisted of my eighty-eight-year-old father and two dads.

I asked myself if this was just a weird coincidence. After all, this was just a small, random group of moms, but the fact that they were experiencing similar feelings of being overwhelmed prompted me to look further. In addition to my clients, I began talking to other moms whenever I could. I asked them if they felt like they had enough time to do all that they needed to on any given day. I talked to them about what stresses them out and what they do to cope. I also drew upon my social work experience recalling the countless families that I had worked with over the years. My conclusion.... moms are stressed and pushed to their physical, mental and emotional limits. It is time to make some changes.

Set the Stage

Tonight, at dinner I took a poll. I asked my husband and kids this question. "Since we have been living in this house how many toilets have you cleaned?" They all looked at me as if this was a trick question. It was really a no-brainer and a simple calculation for each of them. But just for fun, we did the math. Living in this house for eleven years we multiplied the number of toilets by the number of times each toilet is cleaned per week by five-hundred-and-seventy-two weeks. The equation for each of them looked like this zero x zero = zero.

My number was a little different. Given that we have multiple toilets, I multiplied the number of toilets by the number of times I usually clean them per week, then multiplied that by the number of weeks we have lived in our home. Of course, this is a rough estimate but when I did the math it seems that I have cleaned approximately four-thousand-five-hundred-and-seventy-six toilets in the past eleven years.

So that is not a problem except for the fact that no one else has ever cleaned one.... EVER!

The final calculations:

Mom: 4,576 toilets cleaned

Everyone else combined: 0 toilets cleaned

Okay, the kids get a free pass for their younger years, so I expected their number to be low, but they are older now and each of them is fully capable of doing their share. Oh, and let's not forget the forty-eight-year-old, I think he is quite capable, especially given that he gets the most use out of the facilities...just saying.

What is wrong with this picture? I'll tell you what's wrong with this picture...I painted it. That's right, I allowed it to happen. The toilets are just one example, but for years I did everything. I never asked for help with anything, even basic daily household cleaning.

As a nutritional biochemist, international author and speaker, Dr. Libby Weaver explains, "Behavior is the outermost expression of our inner beliefs."[1] In other words, how we behave is rooted in what we believe. I really believed that I was sub-par as a mother and a wife if I couldn't get it all done because it seemed to me that the other moms I knew were sailing through. I no longer believe this. In fact, I believe the opposite. I believe that many moms are just like me, desperately, craving a minute of peace. I believe that I have value and should not serve 24/7 at the expense of my health. I believe that I deserve some downtime (and so do you) which can easily be accomplished with a team effort.

The struggle is real my friends, and it is not one that we should have alone. A good friend once gave me great advice. "Start as you mean to go on," she said to me. Meaning, that it is much harder to change things when they have been done a certain way for a long time. Unfortunately, I did not heed her advice at the time and years later found myself saying 'ah-ha,' that is what she meant.

This is important especially if you are a new wife or mom. Set the stage now. Ask for shared responsibility from your partner now. Trust me, it will be much harder down the road when your spouse is used to you doing everything and you suddenly ask for his (or her) participation. I hate to compare this to training a dog, but well, the comparison seems to fit. If you train your dog to sit when he is a puppy then sitting on command will be second nature to him. If from the time you get married or have kids you and your partner share responsibilities instead of it all falling on one person, it will make a much more harmonious household for everyone involved. There will be no need to feel defeated when you can't do it all because you won't be expected to.

Okay, that was my little tidbit for the new wives or moms who still believe in fairytales;) Now back to the rest of us who are well aware that that ship has sailed, and it is going to take a major storm to get it back to port.

Definitions

My husband was off to do something and I pointed out to him how he puts his leisure activities above all else, including my work. He graciously provided me with an explanation for this. He said that this is how it is supposed to be. I asked him to clarify this statement and he responded by saying that this is what the dictionary definition of 'mom' is. And I quote, "Right next to the word mom in the dictionary it says... to take care of everyone else before yourself."

So, of course, I had to ask, what does it say for dad? His definition of dad? Well, he said it is like the vice president is to the president. In the event the mom cannot fulfill all of her duties, the dad needs to step in, but until then he is in the background handling things like delegating jobs to others or handing out punishments when needed. Really? Are you #$%^&*! kidding me?

He said this half-jokingly but, I stress the word 'half' as I know there is a seed of truth to his statement. I bring this up because while people may not say this out loud, this is what many people believe and expect from their wives, mothers, and grandmothers.

Let's dispel this myth right now. Being a good mother does not mean sacrificing yourself! This bears repeating. Being a good mother does not mean sacrificing yourself! You cannot effectively take care of everyone else without taking care of yourself.

When you get on an airplane the flight attendant explains to the passengers all about safety procedures. The message here is poignant. Before putting an oxygen mask on someone else you must first put one on yourself. Why? Because you can't help other people if you pass out from lack of oxygen. Common sense, right? Right! This applies to daily life as well. You cannot take care of everyone else without taking care of yourself. Eventually, you will crash. So, do yourself and your family a favor and put your oxygen mask on. Taking care of yourself is the best thing you can do for your whole family.

Houston, We Have a problem!

I was working full time, caring for my kids, providing care to my elderly parents, running a household, taxi service, maid service, you know, the works. My job was extremely demanding and not one I ever left, meaning that when I came home, my work came with me in the form of emails, texts, and calls that had to be responded to. There were reports to be read and decisions to be made that - oftentimes had to be done during my family time.

This constant barrage of work left me feeling guilty. I felt guilty when I was at work because I wasn't home with my kids. When I was home, I felt guilty that I wasn't putting more hours in at the office. In addition to the guilt, was the constant thinking about the other. When my kids would tell me something I was really trying to listen, but inevitably my mind would wander to the many things I needed to accomplish at work. When one of my colleagues posed a question, it was the same thing. While I was looking at them, my brain was not always comprehending what they were saying. Instead, I was thinking about which kid had to get to which sport after school and how I could possibly be in three places at once and still get dinner on the table. We have to get homework in there at some point and I have a PTA meeting.... I was not fully present for anything or anyone, including myself. My head was a virtual whirlwind of activity. My life had become one giant To-Do list and nowhere on that list was anything even remotely related to self-care. I was last on the list. Actually, let me correct myself, I was not even on the list. The needs of my kids, my husband, my parents, my clients, my staff, and even virtual strangers came before mine. Knowing that I was only hanging on by a thread I would still volunteer my time for the PTA, little league, networking groups or any other organization I felt obligated to participate in.

I was mom, wife, daughter, caretaker, coach, teacher, director, chauffeur, chef, cleaning lady, dog walker, and the list goes on. But who was I really? I had no clue. When I looked in the mirror, I didn't even recognize the face staring back at me. I had lost myself, lost my identity because every day was only about getting things done. I judged my success on whether everything on my list for that particular day was complete.

There was no depth or substance. My personality had changed. My words were quick and not well thought out. I was annoyed a lot and very easily agitated. I was not the mother I wanted to be, I was not the wife I wanted to be, and I certainly wasn't the person I wanted to be. I was spent, mentally, emotionally and physically. And I was hanging on by a thread.

Internally I would beat myself up because I had no business complaining. I knew I had a lot to be grateful for, so who the hell was I to complain, right? I should be happy, but I wasn't. I was angry and getting angrier all the time. It wasn't material things I was longing for; it was peace and time with my children. It wasn't just time though, and although I hate the term "quality time," dammit, that is what I longed for. I wanted time where we actually took a breath, looked at each other and connected. This is what was missing, and I know I am not alone in this. So many of the women I have spoken to have told me the same thing. They just can't keep up.

Let me set the record straight. If you are among these women there is nothing wrong with you. I repeat there is nothing wrong with you! It is normal (if there is such a thing as normal) to want, no to need, a break. The body and the brain are wired in such a way that refueling is necessary. Our male counterparts do it quite often, at least the ones I know.

You deserve the same thing. When you go from one task to the next without ever taking some time for yourself then the chronic stress response begins. (We'll talk in-depth about that later on) You need quiet or downtime. This should be made a priority. Stress is arguably one of the biggest challenges we face as it can have devastating effects on multiple systems in our body. This is a topic that will come up at various times in this book because it goes hand-in-hand with other topics covered. Along with explaining the effects that stress can have on your body, I will give you practical tools that can help to reduce your stress level and cope with the stress that is unavoidable.

In order to effectively change something, one must identify the problem and actively take steps toward change. So, we have identified a problem. Noticing it and bitching about it doesn't help; believe me, I did this for years. For me, the change did not occur until I let go of my pride and said I need help. Being a very proud woman, this was incredibly difficult for me to do. My warped view of my persona was that of Supermom...I could do it all. My reality was that I could not continue to do it all without serious consequences to my health. I explained to my husband what I had known but ignored for some time, that all of the illnesses I had were my body's way of telling me to make changes. I told him that something was going to give and that something was going to be me.

When I first said this out loud, I felt defeated, a little relieved that it was out there, but still defeated. In my mind, I was a failure. I thought that most moms I know live the same kind of lives and they manage just fine. But the fact of the matter is they aren't managing just fine. They're managing at the expense of themselves just like I had been doing for years.

After taking action, in the form of altering my work schedule and making some changes, I no longer felt like a failure. In fact, I felt empowered. There was another bonus to my actions. I realized that what I did had sent a powerful message to my children, especially my girls. First, they saw me standing up for myself and using my voice to make a change. Secondly, I was modeling for them. I was demonstrating self-care. This was huge because I want them to always make time to take care of themselves. We all know that we can talk with our kids until we are blue in the face about something they should or should not do, but modeling is so much more powerful than any lecture we give them.

They saw their mother standing up for herself and making herself a priority. Now they see that their mom is still taking care of the family but they also continue to see their mother setting boundaries, eating foods that nourish and heal the body, exercising, meditating and practicing Qigong. They see me saying 'no' to outside requests for my time when I know that a yes would require a sacrifice of my time with them or for my own needs. These are the things that I need to do in order to be the best me I can be which translates to a much better mom for them.

This is what worked for me but this is individual. You may have different needs or wants than I did. The key is figuring out exactly what it is you need or want. You have to really look at your own situation and identify what it is that is not working for you.

The Takeaways~

1) Identify your needs (even this can be challenging).

2) Say them out loud.

3) Talk to your family about why it is important that you have your needs met the same way they do.

4) Find an outlet. We will talk more about this later, but it can be one that takes hours, or it can be one that takes five minutes. Hopefully, there will be a little bit of both. A quick-release ...find a quiet spot (I know that is easier said than done) and just take a few deep breaths. You will notice that I have devoted a whole chapter (Nourishing You) to outlets because they are that important.

Address the Medical

Put first things first. It is crucial to get your physical health in check so this is where we will begin. This book is not meant to provide medical advice, but rather serve as a catalyst for conversation with your health care provider as a means to explore what may be ailing you. Several issues I have experienced and that many women I have interviewed have experienced are oftentimes overlooked by mainstream medicine. I will touch on these particular issues in hopes of providing insight on where to begin.

My Story: Parenting in Pain

There are many types of illness and pain. We all experience pain and sickness at one time or another. It may be sporadic or it may be chronic. Regardless of the cause of your pain, the fact is that it is difficult to be a pleasant, happy mom when you are sick or in pain. And when the pain gets really bad it is downright impossible.

Before altering my diet and lifestyle I had daily chronic widespread pain, inflammation, and fatigue. I could have been the damn poster girl for Lyrica. From the time I woke in the morning my day was a challenge. Challenge number one, putting my feet on the floor. Ankles were swollen and feet throbbed but it had to be done so just do it quickly like swallowing terrible food that your dear, old aunt made especially for you. Then there were the hands. Okay, time to straighten the fingers, which were also swollen and a little bent like the hands of someone twice my age. Then there were the hips, the back, the ribs, and the neck. The key was to get moving to reduce some of this pain but a lot of it remained throughout the day.

I saw several doctors in order to try to figure out what was causing my pain. Some took me seriously and others dismissed my complaints. One doctor sarcastically told me that I was very in tune with my body. This was not meant as a compliment. In his eyes, I was just another woman bitching about random pain.

Then there were the docs who found diagnoses for my symptoms. And diagnose they did. I was diagnosed with a whole host of illnesses including Ankylosing Spondylitis, Lyme's Disease, Fibromyalgia, Chronic Fatigue Syndrome and the list goes on. The treatment for every one of my diagnoses was drugs, drugs, and more drugs. There were the anti-inflammatories and the biologics for the AS and of course major long-term, antibiotics to treat the Lyme.

When I was diagnosed with Ankylosing Spondylitis (a severe form of arthritis), I asked the doctor if he was certain that I had this or if it was possible that my inflammation could be caused by something else. He said that he could tell me with one-hundred-percent certainty that this was the correct diagnosis. He also said that the only treatment for me was a monthly biologic injection with a laundry list of possible serious side effects. I was a young mother and I could not risk the side effects associated with this treatment. I asked this particular doctor if there were any foods that might help with the inflammation or exercises that might help me. He chuckled and said with absolute certainty "No. The injections are your only option. If you don't take them you will be crippled by the time you are fifty." I walked out of there feeling very discouraged but still thinking that there had to be some other way.

It is an interesting dynamic when a highly-recommended and very well-respected rheumatologist gives you information, and, in your mind, you are saying to yourself, he is full of shit. I mean who I am to question this expert in his field? I have no training in rheumatology, hell, I have no medical training at all, and still, my inner voice was not quieting down. The voice inside said, 'this can't be right, press on until you get a better answer.' So, press on I did. This time I was going to a top doc in Manhattan. This one didn't feel I needed to start off with the extreme treatment of Enbrel but that if we didn't get it under control, I may end up needing it. He put me on a couple of milder meds to start and was optimistic that with ongoing treatment I could get my pain and swelling controlled. This doc also did not suggest any change in diet but he did recommend that I swim. He suggested that swimming was a great way to increase mobility without the use of drugs. This was good news as I was all about not taking meds if I didn't have to. I am one of those people that always (and I mean always) ends up with one of the side effects listed under "In rare cases." So, I began to swim. Swimming was helpful as it made me feel weightless and took the pressure off of my joints. It gave me some relief, but I was still hurting.

In addition to the joint pain, swelling and overall body pain I constantly got infections. Sinus infections were the norm for me, but over time they got more severe and new types of infections surfaced. Docs just pumped me up with antibiotic after antibiotic. I was on them more than I was off. My body began to build up a resistance to these antibiotics and the infections got worse. First came the repeated staff and strep infections, then MRSA and finally the mother of all infections, Clostridium Difficile aka CDiff. CDiff is a serious intestinal infection, which in many cases is fatal. People with healthy immune systems are usually able to fight off CDiff. When I contracted CDiff, the first-time doctors surmised that it was because I was on antibiotics. After all, when looking at me they saw a healthy young woman so that had to be the reason I contracted this serious illness. The only problem was that I was not on antibiotics at the time and even though they didn't notice, I was far from healthy. After my second bout with CDiff, I thought 'okay, something is seriously wrong with me.' I later learned that I contracted CDiff not from being on antibiotics at the time but that my long-term overuse of antibiotics combined with a poor diet had virtually wiped out my body's natural defenses. All the good bacteria in my gut were gone and my immune system was shot. Someone could have a cold two blocks away and I would catch the damn thing. The problem was I didn't know why, and neither did any of the doctors I saw at the time.

As my issues got worse one of my kids also began having some health problems. We took her to specialist after specialist. Without a definitive diagnosis, she too was offered a plethora of medications to treat symptoms without getting to the cause. Something inside of me was saying no. No to putting a then eleven-year-old girl on birth control pills to get rid of headaches. I said no to another medication prescribed to her that had serious side effects. In my opinion, the risks outweighed the benefits, but doctors who had no answers about her condition were quick to prescribe.

Again, I didn't have medical training, so who was I to say no to these medications that may reduce my daughter's symptoms? I will tell you who I was. I was a mom following her instincts and knowing that there had to be more to this. This was when I decided to head back to school. God helps those who help themselves, I thought. And so, I started my journey toward restoring my health and that of my family.

I started to question everything. Sometimes what I learned ignited more questions. Did I ever have Ankylosing Spondylitis or Fibromyalgia? Looking back, I can honestly say that I don't think so. I began to educate myself and then formally went back to school to earn a certification as a Holistic Health Coach.

Today my inflammation and pain are gone. I did not take biologics to accomplish this. I changed my diet. After doing an elimination diet to see how different types of foods affected me, I learned that gluten and dairy were serious triggers for me. I eliminated these two things from my diet in hopes of addressing the infections, pain, and inflammation but I was pleasantly surprised when other things fell into place as well.

Of course, I was thrilled my pain and inflammation went away and the infections subsided. What I didn't expect was that the severe seasonal allergies I had suffered from since childhood were literally gone. I was no longer tired all the time. I didn't have to carry an inhaler because I could breathe…no more asthma! My headaches were few and far between now. My menstrual cramps were not nearly as bad as they had been for as long as I could remember. And I can't forget the phenomenon called brain fog. Well, it didn't go away completely, but it did improve. I could think more clearly. In addition to changing my diet, I knew by now that I also needed to restore the bacteria in my gut to get back on track. I enlisted the help of an amazing functional medicine doctor who helped me do this the right way and also got my hormones, sleep, and stress in order.

As for my daughter, after years of seeing specialists and searching for answers as to what was making her so sick, we finally got answers. With the help of an incredible doctor who took the time to listen to me and to her, this issue is improving every day. He diagnosed her with SIBO. Her illness was also related to diet and the overuse of antibiotics when she was a young child. As a result of her illness, she had permeation of her intestine a.k.a., leaky gut, which allowed toxins to enter her bloodstream more easily and also interfered with her absorption of essential nutrients. While some medication was necessary to eliminate the overgrowth of bad bacteria in her small intestine, it was that of an herbal variety with no harmful side effects. The elimination of certain foods is a key component of her treatment. It has been a long and difficult road for her, but it has been one with much healing through food and supplements instead of major prescription medications. For this I am grateful.

While you may not have SIBO (although many Americans probably do and don't know it) or Ankylosing Spondylitis, if you are out of balance you probably struggle with some form of illness, inflammation, or chronic health issue. This book is not intended to provide medical advice, but it will give you solid insight into ways of improving your daily life, and in doing so, you should see some positive changes you didn't expect.

East Meets West

"Human felicity is produced not so much by great pieces of good fortune that seldom happen but as by little advantage that occur every day."
Benjamin Franklin

Before you can add on to your house you have to have your foundation poured. Before you can build upon your foundation, that foundation must be solid. If there are any loose bricks it can throw off the whole house. The same holds true with your body. In order to achieve optimal health, you must first have a solid foundation. If anyone system is off it can affect others. This can be a vicious cycle, so getting proper medical treatment is key.

I want to touch on the fact that in some ailments there are options when it comes to medical care. In addition to traditional, Western medical care, seeing a functional medicine doctor, naturopath or a practitioner that practices Eastern medicine can be advantageous.

Just a quick note on the differences between the two. Western medicine sees the mind and body as two separate entities, which do not intersect. This is the primary form of care that is typically used in the United States. Western medicine can be life-saving and is often necessary. That being said, it has been my experience that some western medicine practitioners tend to jump right to the prescription meds without identifying the root cause of the problem. These are well intentioned practitioners but the training the receive is usually that of a disease-based model rather than a patient focused approach. Oftentimes this means the symptoms are treated without identifying or treating the cause. And let's face it, with the emergence of managed care, even the most caring doctor is limited in terms of the time, energy and resources he or she can devote to a single patient.

Some Eastern practices, such as Chinese or Ayurvedic medicine, have a different approach. Eastern medicine sees the mind and body as one connected system. It takes a 'whole person approach' and focuses on identifying the source of a problem. Functional medicine works the same way. For some people, treatment of an ailment may be as simple as a change in diet and lifestyle, manipulation of the body's energy or the supplementation of certain vitamins or trace minerals.

Whenever possible I want to eliminate the problem at its source rather than putting a temporary band-aid over it. To me, this just makes the most sense. Both of these styles of practice have great value and the truth is you don't have to choose between them. You can put the two together and get the best of both worlds.

The Institute for Functional Medicine provides information as well as being a good tool to help you find a practitioner in your area.

https://www.functionalmedicine.org/practitioner

The Doctor-Patient Relationship: Finding a good fit

The doctor-patient relationship should be a team effort. You both bring something valuable to the table. Your doctor has medical expertise and years of training. You are the expert on you: you have years of training on how your body functions and responds. Even if you don't have a name for it, you know when something is not quite right with your body. Do your homework and find a doctor or health care provider who will take the time to listen to what you have to say. You will know it is a good fit when you feel comfortable in bringing any and all information to him or her without fear of being judged or rushed. Don't be afraid to ask for clarification, to question, or even to disagree with your doctor. Ultimately your treatment is your decision. A second or even third opinion might be what you need to ensure you are making the best possible decision for you.

A few years ago, I had terrible pain in my elbow and saw an orthopedist. He took an X-ray and noted an issue. He started by giving me anti-inflammatory medication and a brace to wear. Then came injections of cortisone. When this did not relieve my symptoms, he suggested that he could operate to fix the problem. Having had success with physical therapy for other issues, I asked if this would be an option. He said I could try it. He said he didn't originally suggest it because as a working mom, he didn't think I would have the time to put into it. I let him know that I was not ready to jump into surgery but I was in enough pain to make the time for PT. So off I went to my PT evaluation. The physical therapist spent a good amount of time asking me questions and then got to the physical exam. Throughout the process, she explained each step to me and to her intern who was very lucky to be learning from this talented woman. Within minutes she had identified a problem. She asked me to turn my head and manipulated my arm. While there was still a little soreness, the intense pain was instantly gone. She explained that a bone was out of place and simply needed to be put back into place. She advised that I would need a few sessions of PT to build up my strength due to the fact I had not been able to use the arm for months. Done, fixed without surgery! Had I not questioned the doctor I would have unnecessarily gone under the knife and had a long, drawn-out recovery. Talk about a time sucker!

Takeaways:

1- You should be looked at as a partner in your health care. After all, it is your health care, right? Any doctor that dismisses your input is doing you a disservice.
2- Be your own advocate. Don't be afraid to question a doctor or medical professional if what they are saying doesn't make sense to you.

Clean up the Endocrine

Did you know that hormones affect every organ in your body? The endocrine system is a group of glands that produces various hormones. In addition to other functions, these hormones are responsible for regulating metabolism, mood, sleep, reproduction, and sexual function. Getting this system operating at its best is crucial to maintaining good physical and mental health.

I recommend a thorough medical check-up to ensure that all systems in your body are working properly. Many of you are probably saying ugh, who has time for this. To this I say, make the time. Think of this as bringing your car to get checked out before a long road trip. Yes, another metaphor: You want to make sure every part of your car is working properly so it can go the distance and get you to your destination safely. Well, guess what, your body is your 'car' in life. You want it to serve you well for the long haul and not break down. When one system is out of whack it can and often does impact other systems in your body. For example, if your hormones are out of balance it can affect your sleep patterns and when you don't sleep well your cognitive function can be impaired and when your cognitive function is impaired you have less patience and can make poor decisions. It can be a vicious cycle, so getting a handle on it as early as possible is key.

My husband lovingly refers to me as vertically challenged. I often respond with 'small but mighty.' This is the perfect description of the pituitary gland. It sits at the base of the brain under the hypothalamus and is a tiny, but powerful gland responsible for producing hormones that control other parts of the endocrine system. It is governed by the hypothalamus. The hypothalamus serves as a liaison between the nervous system and the endocrine system. Why is this important? Because it is all connected, and as I said, if one part of the system is off it can throw off the whole show.

A thorough check-up of the function of the endocrine system is especially important for women because our bodies are always changing, so having hormone levels where they need to be is crucial. Making sure that the thyroid and adrenal glands are functioning properly is at the top of the list, as thyroid and cortisol imbalances are not uncommon. These hormonal changes can account for many different challenges you may be facing such as weight gain, cravings, irritability, insomnia, poor concentration, and many other conditions. In addition to traditional medical care, I especially recommend seeing a functional medicine doctor or a practitioner that practices holistic medicine, in order to have a thorough check-up in this department.

To get an idea of how a gland malfunctioning can throw off your body let's look at the thyroid gland. The thyroid is responsible for regulating metabolism. If your thyroid function is off it can affect your energy level, your weight, and your body temperature just to name a few.

Hyperthyroidism (overactive thyroid) is associated with weight loss, rapid or irregular heartbeat, fatigue, muscle weakness, increased appetite, anxiety and irritability, excessive sweating, sleep problems, and the list goes on. Symptoms of Hypothyroidism (underactive thyroid) include fatigue, weakness, irritability, feeling cold, becoming forgetful, weight gain, hair loss, depression, and decreased libido. And I am only scratching the surface with those I just listed. Issues with the thyroid can wreak havoc on your ability to function. Many Western medicine doctors seem to only examine TSH and T4 but looking at free T4, free T3, and reverse T3 (rT3) levels are needed for a complete picture.[1] Most functional medicine doctors will do a complete panel. Regulating your thyroid will make a world of difference in the way you feel.

Balancing sex hormones is another important task at hand. Common female hormonal imbalances are low progesterone, high estrogen or estrogen dominance, low estrogen, low androgens, and excess androgens. I won't get into this too much but please note that each of these imbalances has a whole host of physiological issues associated with them. The bottom line is that any of the imbalances mentioned above will make you feel like shit in one way or another.

Just to give one example, let's look at low progesterone. Just a side note for you to know when reviewing results with your doc... Progesterone is measured in relation to how much estrogen a person has. There are many roles that progesterone plays including the regulation of mood. Low progesterone can contribute to heavy periods, menstrual migraines, PMS or PMDD, difficulty getting and staying pregnant, abdominal bloating and changes in mood. *Did I mention mood?* Yeah, that was a big one for me. Yes, I know I am being repetitive here but I think this bears repeating as mood is an issue for a lot of women. Progesterone helps to regulate mood. Anyone out there having any issues with that one? Well here's where it gets good. As I said before, it's all connected. Low progesterone can be caused by high cortisol. (Cortisol is a stress hormone produced in the adrenal gland) When someone is chronically stressed progesterone production takes a back seat.

Cortisol is what I consider the smoking gun and it is often overlooked by mainstream medicine. According to Dr. Josh Axe, "Chronic, high cortisol production is tied to symptoms and ailments including weight gain, anxiety, sleep disorders, hormonal imbalances and fertility problems, in addition to many other problems."[2]

While cortisol has an important role, for many it is overproduced or underproduced as a result of chronic stress. This can lead to a condition called

HPA (Hypothalamus Pituitary Adrenal)-axis Dysfunction.

> "The stress response is primarily governed by the hypothalamic–pituitary–adrenal (HPA) axis. Stress activates the HPA axis and sets off a cascade of neuroendocrine signals that ultimately leads to the release of hormones and neurotransmitters like cortisol, norepinephrine (noradrenaline), and epinephrine (adrenaline). Over time, the chronic activation of our stress–response system erodes resilience and depletes metabolic reserve. Resilience is the immediate capacity of cells, tissues, and organ systems to respond to changes in physiological needs. Metabolic reserve refers to the long-term capacity of our body to respond to these changes. The loss of resilience and the depletion of metabolic reserve lead to changes in cortisol output (most commonly too much, but sometimes too little), disruption of the diurnal cortisol rhythm (too little cortisol in the morning or too much at night), and changes in the production of other hormones and neurotransmitters related to the HPA axis, such as DHEA, melatonin, and epinephrine." [3]

This is another reason that ensuring healthy adrenal function is key. With all of my medical issues, not one traditional doctor examined my adrenal function or hormone levels, even though many of my symptoms screamed of issues in this department. It wasn't until I saw a functional medicine doctor that this was addressed and my life changed almost instantly. I stopped waking up in the middle of the night with my heart racing. My anxiety lessened and I was not wound so tight. This was huge for me. Please ask your doctor to check your adrenal function. Having your cortisol levels regulated can change your life. It did mine. If your traditional medical care isn't addressing the endocrine, please consider finding a practitioner who practices whole-body medicine. In a nutshell, if your hormones are off so are you! Remember the oxygen mask.... you first!

Meet Raven

June 21, 2017 - I wake up with my heart racing and my head pounding, feeling kind of shaky. Bloated and crampy doesn't begin to describe the abdominal pain I'm experiencing. My vision is blurry, I feel nauseous and the light hurts my eyes. Every sound echoes through my head like there are amplifiers in my ears. All I want to do is shut off the lights, take something for the pain, and go back to bed; but I can't. I am Mom and everyone depends on me. So, I drag myself out of bed and start doing what needs to be done for my family. I know these symptoms mean my period is close. I want it to come so I can go back to feeling human again.

The last two days, I have been like a ticking time bomb: anything will set me off. To describe my disposition, well let's see…moody doesn't quite cut it…. on edge… yup the sharpest edge you can find…. irritable, well yes, but that is way too nice. Okay, let's just say it like it is. I am a raging bitch for these two-to-three days a month. They call our period 'our friend.' Well, my friend is a full-fledged witch. That's right, I have an inner witch that makes her presence known on these days each month. I like to call her Raven. When Raven shows up everything pisses me off, even the normal stuff. If the kids fight, I'm yelling at them. If my husband asks me about something, I have explained to him three times already, then lookout. He is going to get an earful about how he doesn't listen to a word I say…ever! He may even have to sit through me ranting about something he did ten years ago, but oh well, Raven is in town. And if the timing of Raven's visit happens to be on the rare occasion when my mother-in-law comes to visit, there can be rage of epic proportions. That combination is unequivocally the perfect storm! If the regular things in life bother me in this state, well then you can imagine the fury that lies within when a virtual stranger comes to my home telling me what I should do differently, and how lucky I am to have married her son. Occasionally, I was able to internally reason with Raven and talk her off the proverbial ledge. For the most part, I would just utilize my quick wit to respond to my mother-in-law's comments with a joke or sarcastic statement that she was unsure how to take, but my poor husband heard about it later. Then again, my poor husband should be standing up to his mommy's Raven;)

When Raven was in town, situations I would usually have some patience for were fair game. For example, if I was driving and someone cut me off, let's just say the reaction would be totally different if it happened on day twenty-six of my cycle instead of day six.

In addition to the mental symptoms, I was having a lot of physical symptoms as well, which just added insult to injury. These symptoms included extremely painful periods, migraines, and I was bleeding like I needed triage every month.

The answers came when I finally dragged myself to a functional medicine doctor. Mind you I was going to her for a whole host of issues not related to my menstrual cycle. The fact that she figured this out for me was an added bonus that I did not expect, but in her thorough and comprehensive approach to health care, she has discovered so much that has improved my overall quality of life.

So, bottom line …I am not a raving lunatic. It wasn't me or my personality. My emotional rants were happening because my hormones were severely out of balance. If you are experiencing any of this, there is hope, and there is help. For me, it came in the form of some supplements, diet change, daily meditation, and breathwork. I'm not talking hours in solitude saying ohm. Just give yourself five minutes a day to do a quick meditation or breathwork or both. We'll talk more about that later.

Today my periods are not a problem. I very rarely even get cramps but if I do it is nothing crazy. My painful ovarian cysts have resolved. If I get a headache, it is just a headache, not a migraine, but even headaches are becoming rare. I no longer need a mop and bucket for the crazy heavy bleeding. As for Raven, let's just say I can keep her in check. I no longer feel like a raving lunatic on the days just before my period. Listen, I'm no Mary Poppins and my inner witch is still there, (just a little;) but I control her instead of the other way around which I'm sure my family appreciates as much as I do.

The caveat here is not to let your voice be pigeonholed into a Raven-rant when others want to discredit your words:)

The Takeaway ~ If you are experiencing any of the symptoms I described, see a doctor. As I mentioned earlier, my preference is a Functional Medicine Doctor or Naturopath, as they tend to go deeper than the surface to get to the root cause of the problem and offer a lot of natural solutions. There is help out there and you may be pleasantly surprised at how much better you can feel.

Brain Fog

Brain Fog, simply put, is that feeling that you can't keep your thoughts straight. You are forgetting things, getting confused, feeling lethargic. I hate to admit it, but this was the worst of what was holding me back.

While there are varying degrees of Brain Fog, mine was pretty severe and getting worse all the time. For years I chalked it up to having an attention deficit. For as long as I can remember I have a major problem with focus and concentration. I struggled in high school because I would read something several times and still have no idea what I just read. My inability to focus got worse as time went on. It wasn't until my mid-thirties that I realized this was becoming a major problem but it wasn't until several years after that when I finally acknowledged it and began looking for answers. It's the same old story though…Mom's stuff on the back burner. The others need me and they come first. In the meantime, my problem got worse.

There were times when I thought there was something seriously wrong with my brain. Why couldn't I think straight? Why couldn't I comprehend? Even trying to help my kids with homework was difficult. I couldn't recall history and don't even get me started on the math. I was frustrated and embarrassed.

I felt stupid, however on another level I felt like a genius as I was able to fake my way through just about everything in life, work, school, and social situations. I could hold my own in a debate over politics and important issues, but I couldn't remember what my co-worker said to me two minutes ago. It was crazy. Here I was with a Bachelor's Degree, a Master's Degree and a considerable amount of postgraduate work, and I felt like I knew absolutely nothing.

I wondered if I had a cognitive disorder, which really worried me. I mean, put my memory problems together with a family history of mental illness and dementia and now I was shitting the proverbial brick. As with so many other things, I still did not make this a priority, but while seeing my primary care doctor for a more serious issue I mentioned my memory problems to him.

He suggested an MRI of my brain just to be on the safe side. When the MRI came back showing several legions of white matter on my brain, he referred me to a neurologist. Okay, now this sounded bad. What the hell was wrong with me? My doctor reassured me that this was probably nothing to worry about but out of his scope so off to the neurologist, I went. The neurologist told me there was nothing to be concerned about but that this white matter could be indicative of another issue so I was sent for more testing. Nothing earth-shattering was revealed but in the process of this testing, I was told that I was positive for Lyme's Disease so since there was no other reason for the white matter, Lyme was assumed to be the cause.

The doctor I saw for the Lyme's suggested that I try temporarily eliminating wheat from my diet to help with my joint inflammation. That did reduce the inflammation but guess what else seemed to improve...my concentration. There was an instant improvement, but definitely not a total fix. There were more subtle and gradual changes over the course of the next several years. Around this time, I began my course of study and learned of the connection between gluten and something called brain fog. I would also come to learn that white matter showing up on an MRI is indicative of gluten sensitivity.[1] It all made sense now. Well at least after reading it five or six times:)

So, there was a significant improvement now that I was gluten-free. However, significant for me was still not great. My mother had been diagnosed with dementia and I thought that perhaps my memory loss was a precursor to what I thought might be my fate as well. It was better, but I was still forgetting and getting confused and not comprehending things that I should. There was another piece to this puzzle and this is why I can't stress enough the importance of functional medicine. My functional medicine doctor started questioning me about my sleep. Turns out that lack of sleep, or even regularly disrupted sleep, can have catastrophic effects on your memory. So as not to be redundant I won't go into detail about sleep now as I cover that in the sleep chapter but suffice it to say improving my sleep was huge when it came to improving my memory.

The final piece was fats. There was a period of time in my youth when I believed what I heard without examining the source of the information. During this time there was one major media fallacy that I adhered to ...eliminating fat from my diet. I fell hook line and sinker for the whole fat-free craze, thinking it would help me achieve optimum health, I eliminated fats from my diet. I increased carbs, you know the kind ...the fat-free cookies and crackers loaded with chemicals and sugar, that we were made to believe were a healthy option. I would later come to learn of the important role that good fats have in the diet, especially for brain health. In doing without significant fat in my diet for a good two years I believe I may have done some damage to my brain. That is a strong statement but one I believe wholeheartedly. There is good news though. According to renowned neurologist, Dr. David Perlmutter, brain cells can be regenerated and that we have some control over this process with diet and lifestyle. [2] I am thrilled to say that I have seen tremendous improvements in my cognitive abilities with the removal of gluten, prioritizing of sleep and the addition of healthy fats to my diet.

The Takeaway~ Barring any medical issues affecting your brain, a general sense of brain fog can be improved. I urge you to look at the three things that have helped me and countless others in this area.

1- Try eliminating gluten. You may be pleasantly surprised at what you find. This simple step can open a virtual Pandora's box of positive effects on your body. For some, inflammation goes away or their autoimmune disease suddenly improves or resolves. For others, it may be weight loss or the resolution of IBS or acne or maybe just doing a lot less random farting.

2- Sleep, Sleep, Sleep! I can't stress enough the importance of sleep on your body and its ability to regenerate all of its systems, especially brain cells and function.

3- Eat your fats! Healthy fats are essential to brain function. Without them, your brain cannot do its job

Self-Acceptance

Own It

"To be beautiful means to be yourself. You don't need to be accepted by others. You need to accept yourself." ~Zen Master Thich Nhat Hanh

Self-acceptance is very liberating. It takes a lot of unnecessary stress away, and let's face it, we have enough stress already without a lack of self-acceptance. We should all celebrate who we are: big, small, fat, skinny, big-boned, dark, light, or whatever. This is not to say that we should not make changes to improve our health, but we need to start owning who we are.

Have you ever heard someone say, "She has no business wearing that?" The funny thing is every time I have heard this statement it came from a woman. It is usually said because the woman she is referring to is heavy or has a lot of curves. What makes it okay for a skinny girl to wear a bikini but not a full-figured woman? My answer is 'nothing.'

I have to throw in my health coach disclaimer here, which is that being extremely overweight or underweight can have health risks. As such, I encourage people to get a regular physical and address any medical issues. If you are having trouble with losing or gaining weight, to get yourself to a healthy weight for you, again I recommend seeing a functional medicine doctor or naturopath who can assess if there are issues with digestion or assimilation.

Now back to the matter at hand. As long as you have addressed your possible medical issues, you need to be the 'you' that makes you happy. I repeat the 'you' that makes *YOU* happy.

A faulty message has been delivered to women and girls for decades. Unfortunately, the media's depiction of beauty is a very limited view and the motivation behind it is selling products. Their disproportionate ideal is not even real without surgery, enhancements or photo-doctoring. These warped messages about how women should look are par for the course. Messages of how girls should look start at a very young age and can have devastating effects.

I took my daughter to buy her new jeans when she was ten years old. Now by no means was she a skinny kid, but she wasn't overweight either. She was athletic and I used to refer to her as solid. At no time did her pediatrician say that she needed to lose weight because she didn't. Well, skinny jeans were everywhere and this simply was not an option for her. There were no local stores that carried jeans for a girl with her proportions. Let me just reiterate that her proportions were not abnormal. Even with an extensive Internet search, at the time

I was only able to find jeggings that looked like jeans that she could wear.

This is a problem. What kind of message does this send to a ten-year-old girl? It tells her she is outside of the norm if she can't even find one pair of jeans to fit her in mainstream stores. It also tells her that if you want to wear the 'cool' clothes you have to be super thin. But there were plenty of girls her size in the same boat. They were at a healthy weight but could not find clothes that were in style to fit. And so, it begins, the message conveyed to our girls that they must change themselves to be accepted. We must all work to debunk these fallacies.

The fact is that we are all built differently and we are all beautiful. Our girls need to know this and we need to model it for them. We need to become more comfortable in our own skin. In doing so they will become more comfortable in theirs. If they constantly hear us saying that we are too fat they will become judgmental of their own physical features.

It is easy for me to say 'accept yourself' but is it easy for you to do? Probably not. It wasn't for me at first either and there are still some things with which I struggle. It is a process and it can be work, but believe me when I say it is worth the effort. When you look at yourself from a positive perspective, things start to change.

I believe that while we are all different, we all hold the same intrinsic value. Let me say that again... all people have the same intrinsic value. This is important because we women tend to beat ourselves up over what we could be or think we should be, especially when it comes to our physical features. Again, this is not our fault, we were programmed, but nonetheless, we need to break the cycle.

We can start by simply recognizing that our physical features do not define us. You are amazing just as you are. Rather than getting up in the morning, looking in the mirror and seeing what you don't like, try to start each day taking notice of something you do like about yourself. One thing…anything. Also, take note of something positive about the women around you at least once each day. Once you find one thing you like, you will begin to find more in yourself and in others.

This simple exercise helps us to embrace our differences and recognize how these differences are what make us special. This is the first step toward self-acceptance. Self -acceptance leads to self-love and self-care and that's where we need to be. Remember, in order to take care of others we must take care of ourselves first.

So, go ahead and own who you are. Be proud of who you are and don't let anyone tell you that you are less than amazing. Own it all ...the physical, the mental, the spiritual and even the parts that you consider as defects. These are all the parts of who you are that make you uniquely you, and you are awesome! Believe me, my friends, owning who you are will set you free.

The Internal Conflict

"The noblest art is that of making others happy."
~ PT Barnum

I got up super early this morning so I would have time to write in peace. Working from home can be quite challenging because your work gets overlooked. After all, you are present and therefore available to serve. My family may see writing as my recreation because I enjoy it but it is also my work so I need to designate time to do it.

The fact is that I have to write before everyone wakes up, when no one is home or if all else fails after everyone else has gone to bed. The problem with doing it when everyone is in bed is that by that time, I am exhausted.

What I have just described I am sure you can all relate to, whether you work outside the home, from home or what I like to call 'For the home.' I have done all three of these and at times more than one at a time, as many moms do.

What some may call not working, I call working 'for the home.' Let me first give you my definition of home. It is family, it is food and it is a place where values are instilled and life lessons take place. It should be a safe place where ideas and opinions can be expressed freely and even debated. It should be a place where laughter reigns supreme and children feel the presence of those who love them. Creating and maintaining such a place is hard work. You are the Chief Executive Officer of this vital operation. So, Ms. or Mrs. Jones consider yourself the CEO of Jones Enterprises. You have earned this title!

I think we, as a society, have lost our way a bit as it seems that if there is no dollar sign attached to what we do with our time then the general consensus is that there is no value to it. In my opinion, nothing can be further from the truth. When you give of yourself, there is tremendous value to that. And make no mistake about it, working for the home, being a homemaker, a domestic engineer, a stay-at-home-mom or whatever you want to call it is giving of yourself. In fact, it is an endless giving of yourself. When this is your path, there is no quitting time, no personal days and no sick or vacation benefits.

You are on the clock twenty-four hours a day, seven days per week. This job does not involve lying on the couch with our feet up eating Bonbons.

Yes, being the caretaker of other human beings is a full-time job. Caring for and shaping the lives of other people is arguably one of the most important, if not the most important, job in the world. Yet it is probably the most overlooked and undervalued job in our society.

When I worked outside my home, I felt like others judged me for not being home with my kids. I heard one mom say, "I had to choose between work and kids and I chose my kids." Even though it could not be further from the truth, I felt like she was implying that I chose work over family. Sometimes I would just get this look of pity from a stay-at-home-mom or a comment like, "Oh you work so you must miss a lot." It was like a knife through my heart.

Was I reading too much into comments? Was this my own paranoia about my choices? I wasn't sure so I set out to find some answers. I talked to countless moms and guess what, I am not alone, my friends. Whether we work in or out of the home, many of us struggle with this internal guilt that we should be doing it the other way.

Now my circumstances have changed and I am not working outside of the home. Recently someone said to me, "Oh you don't work? That must be nice." What the hell was she talking about? I do work. I work my ass off. I just don't get paid for it. Instead of saying that or saying nothing, I found myself trying to justify my existence to this person who has no significance in my life. I told her how I am caring for my kids and my sick parents and taking classes and I am starting to write a book. Once she heard that I was sure to get her approval. But why? Why did I want it? I know that taking care of my family is important. Why did I need the external validation of a virtual stranger? I will tell you why. Because we moms have had the seed planted a long time ago that we must do it all. At a very young age, girls are given the message you can have it all: a job, care for your family, do volunteer work, and still have a social life.

Don't get me wrong, this is a great message, it just lacks one thing. Young girls should absolutely know that they can choose their own path. The problem is that with the exception of a family role model, there aren't many messages that recognize or validate the role of a stay-at-home-mom. There are also no media messages that I am aware of that say, 'hey choose your career, get married and have kids because when you have a husband or partner you share the childcare and household duties fifty-fifty.' Yes, ladies, you too can have a full partner in the responsibilities of the home.

Is that message out there? Did I miss it? No, it doesn't exist because, for the most part, the expectation is still that these duties all belong to women.

I am dating myself now but I remember a television commercial from when I was younger. It was a woman all done up in a nice dress singing, " I can bring home the bacon, fry it up in a pan and never let him forget he's a man, cause I'm a woman..." Talk about powerful media messages. This was saying, yes ladies, go out to work, take care of your home and family, and don't forget to please your man.

How about taking care of yourself? Oops, they forgot that. I'm sure it was just an oversight ;) Sure we can have it all, but at what cost? If having it all means never stopping, it will come with a hefty price tag...our health.

Takeaway~ Going to work outside the home or working from home for a salary to help support your family is valuable. Staying home to be a caretaker or working for the home is just as valuable. Some of us have a choice in what we want to do and others don't. Own your role, and do the best you can with the tools you have. Don't lose yourself to the pressures of society to be anything other than who you are. Value yourself and recognize that your role as a mother is significant and important regardless of semantics. When you own it and take pride in your role, again you are sending a powerful message to your children.

Parenting

I am not going to claim to be an expert on parenting. God knows I am not and I don't even feel like I get it right a lot of the time. But here is what I do know. We do the best we can with the tools we are given. So, here's the thing, we all have a different set of tools. When it comes to parenting, it is a constant learning process. We can all stand to sharpen our skillset and seek out new tools, but at the end of the day beating yourself up over what you lack is counterproductive and it will set you back instead of moving you forward.

Owning who you are intrinsically is key. Again, that is not to say that we shouldn't strive for improvement in certain areas, but we must find a way to come to terms with who we are. Doing this can be difficult as it involves accepting that we are flawed. We are intrinsically good but each and every one of us is flawed. Accepting our own unique strengths, weaknesses, and flaws is a challenge, but it is also extremely liberating.

It was probably my greatest epiphany when I realized that in accepting myself, I am teaching my children to accept themselves. That's right, when we reach a place of self-acceptance an amazing thing happens, our children see it. Remember, we are always modeling for our kids whether we realize it or not. They are like little sponges, taking it all in. This means that when they see us beat ourselves up, they are likely to do the same thing. It also means that when they see us accepting ourselves, they are likely to accept who they are and be a little kinder to themselves.

We want our kids to accept themselves and feel good in their own skin. I say to my kids, be the best you that you can be. Stressing the word, *you*. You are who you are and you are intrinsically awesome! I hope that this message will resonate with them. So many kids (and adults) make bad choices simply because they long to fit in or feel accepted. If they feel unconditional acceptance at home and they accept themselves as they are then I believe they will be more inclined to stay true to themselves and not follow the crowd in order to fit in.

The Takeaway~ Accept yourself! Do the best you can with the tools you have and hope to add a tool or two to your tool bag along the way.

Speak Your Truth

"To share your weakness is to make yourself vulnerable; to make yourself vulnerable is to show your strength." — Crissi Jami

The first step into actualizing your female power is to speak your truth. What do I mean by this? Be who you are and don't try to be someone you are not. Say what you mean and mean what you say. Sounds simple enough right? It isn't though …until it is.

As a society, we tend to say what we think people want to hear. But what if we didn't? As women, we are so used to bending over backwards for everyone else that we can really lose ourselves in the mix. Speaking your truth means stepping up and saying to hell with what people think, this is who I am and this is what I need.

Try to just let go. Let go of preconceived notions of who you are, who people think you are, or who people expect you to be. If this is not the real you, I say kiss her goodbye.

This is not easy but I promise you that when you do this you will feel a sense of freedom like nothing you have felt before. When you truly own who you are and accept yourself, warts and all, then you are completely free. You are free of the unnecessary stress of trying to change yourself. Let's face it, that is a lot of work and it is a heavy burden to carry. You can be you, not the you that you want other people to see, the *you* that is real.

When I was a little girl, my teacher told my parents I never raised my hand or spoke in class. My father asked me why that was. I told him I was afraid of being wrong and being made fun of. He looked at me and said, "You shouldn't be afraid to speak up, what you should be afraid of is never being heard." He taught me that my voice was a powerful tool that had great value and that what I had to say was just as important as what anyone else had to say. He taught me it takes great strength to speak from the heart.

That is the message I want to convey to all of you. There is so much value in your voice, your real voice as it represents your true self. I am sure you have heard people say to be true to yourself, but exactly what does that mean? Of course, it means being true to our core values and principles, but I believe it is much more than that. It is listening and trusting your own inner voice. It is putting yourself out there. Again, not the you that you think people want, but the real *you*.

When we use our voices and show our authentic selves to the world, we allow ourselves to be vulnerable. To allow ourselves to be vulnerable is an insanely courageous thing to do. It takes guts and it is risky. But what is the risk to us? Rejection. Will the world appreciate or understand the real me? Maybe but maybe not. You have to be okay with the 'maybe not' outcome and remember that without risk there is no reward. I believe it is better to put the real you forward than a fake version of yourself you use just to appease others. If we do this then we become prisoners, enslaved to an image we create and struggle to maintain.

If we take down any facade and make ourselves vulnerable, the likelihood of developing or improving relationships is terrific. The more real you are the more you will connect with people. Vulnerability is the foundation of self-confidence because once you own your fears and embrace them, you are grounded in the strength of truth. You gain the knowledge that no matter what life throws your way, you can and *will* handle it. [1]

There were a lot of years that I spent trying to be the person I thought I should be. This was not the person I was, or even who I wanted to be. This has changed and I can't even begin to tell you how liberating it is. These days I don't have a problem speaking my truth or using my voice but on the rare occasion that that fear pops up again, I hear my father's words and sometimes John Mayer's too ☺

"*Even if your hands are shaking*
And your faith is broken
Even as the eyes are closing
Do it with a heart wide open say what you need to say, say what you need to say."[2]

I invite you to join me in using your voice and speaking your truth. As a very wise man once said, "*And the truth shall set you free,* "~ Jesus in John 8:32

Stress

Stress is arguably one of the biggest challenges we face and it can have a devastating effect on multiple systems in our body simultaneously. This is a topic that goes hand-in-hand with other topics we've covered. Along with explaining the effects, stress can have on your body I will give you practical tools that can help reduce your stress level. Keep in mind that regardless of changes you make in diet and exercise if you don't find a way to manage your stress you will suffer.

Stress & Your Body

I am sure you have heard too much stress is bad for you. But do you know why? There seems to be a taboo in blaming physical symptoms on stress. It is almost as if doing that has a connotation of weakness, but I am here to tell you that this is simply not the case. There are real physiological changes that occur in the body when a person is constantly experiencing stress.

I think it is important to give a quick overview of these changes since chronic stress affects so many people.

Within our autonomic nervous system, we have the Sympathetic Nervous System and the

Parasympathetic nervous system. The Sympathetic nervous system is utilized in times of stress while the Parasympathetic Nervous System puts the body in a state of rest and allows it to repair itself and refuel. Both systems have vital roles to play in keeping us healthy, but when the SNS is overutilized and the PNS is underutilized, as is the case when we are chronically stressed, we lack the balance and restorative state that we need. So, let's talk about why this is important.

When the brain communicates to the body that there is a threat of danger, the body utilizes the fight or flight response. In order 'to protect us, both our sympathetic nervous system and the endocrine system jump into action.

Hundreds of years ago a threat of danger meant a predator, something like an approaching lion. As humans evolved, so did our lifestyle and perception of what constitutes a stressful situation. Although now there are fewer physical dangers in day-to-day life, that fight or flight mechanism still exists but is often the result of psychological stressors. These psychological stressors vary from person to person, as each person perceives stress differently. Interacting with your boss may elicit the stress response for you while for me it may happen when my newly-licensed son gets behind the wheel of a car.

While we all have different triggers, for many of us these psychological stressors happen frequently, leading to a chronic and habitual stress response within our bodies. This can translate to the overuse of our body's systems and hormones, throwing everything out of whack.

Psychological stress equates to the same rush as a physical threat, except that when it is psychological you experience stress without having that physical outlet that your body expects to follow, which is to run or fight. If there is no physical outlet accompanying the stressful situation, then the body has no way to utilize the stress hormones. This means it has to change the play and adapt. The body says hold up, this isn't how it is supposed to work, and it then has to adapt to these changes and figure out what to do with the extra stress hormones that were not utilized.

Many modern-day situations tend to activate the sympathetic nervous system so let's take a look at what can happen when we constantly activate the Sympathetic Nervous System.

Stress & Illness

According to Dr. Mark Hyman, "When you're stressed, your adrenal glands release hormones like adrenaline and cortisol that flood your system, raising your heart rate, increasing your blood pressure, making your blood more likely to clot, damaging your brain's memory center, increasing belly fat storage and generally wreaking havoc on your body." [1]

The experts at Harvard Medical School state that, the stress response also suppresses the immune system, increasing susceptibility to colds and other illnesses, and the build-up of stress can contribute to anxiety and depression. [2]

Chronic Stress Response & the Endocrine System

When the body is in a constant state of stress, the adrenal glands can get overworked and fail to keep up with the demands being put upon them. This can result in HPA axis dysfunction, which is more commonly referred to as adrenal fatigue. While this is a controversial diagnosis, the belief is that this occurs when the adrenal system gets overworked and eventually slows down. The adrenal glands stop producing hormones efficiently, which throws our hormones out of whack. When this happens, other bodily functions are also affected.

Stress & Important Processes

When our bodies produce stress hormones,

everything we have is focused on saving our lives. Remember the body still thinks it is fending off a lion. Our blood supply, oxygen, and nutrients are sent to our arms and legs in order to give us the power we need to run or fight. As such, what the body considers to be non-essential processes are compromised and do not receive the love and attention they need.

So, this may not be a big deal if it is happening occasionally, but when we experience a chronic stress response these areas suffer. Among these are our skin, hair, and nails. That's right, it can mean your skin loses that glow, your hair can thin and nails become brittle. In my opinion, the most crucial process that becomes neglected in a state of chronic stress is digestion. You may be saying, but this is an essential process and you would be right, but when there is a perceived threat of immediate life-threatening danger, it takes a back seat. Let's face it, we can worry about digesting our food after we fend off the lion. This poses a huge problem for people who are chronically stressed, as poor digestion can open a virtual Pandora's box of illness and chronic health problems.

Stress & Fat

When the Sympathetic Nervous System is activated, the body also reaches for the fastest burning fuel to quickly get it out of the danger that it perceives. This means that when in a constant state of stress, the body is constantly utilizing glucose storage instead of burning fat for fuel. So being constantly stressed may contribute to some extra weight especially around the middle.

Internationally Acclaimed Nutritional Biochemist, Author and Speaker, Dr. Libby Weaver states, "Continual overproduction of cortisol (our long-term stress hormone) can lead to visceral fat gain, the type located inside our abdomen that is strongly linked to inflammation and an increased risk of many diseases." [3]

Stress & Sleep

Ever heard the saying I sleep with one eye open? This is essentially what is happening when you are stressed. As a means of protecting you from that perceived threat, adrenaline keeps you from going into that deep sleep that your body desperately needs to repair itself. After all, you need to be able to jump into action when the lion gets close!

To recap, the parasympathetic nervous system is where we need to be to recharge and heal. When the sympathetic nervous system is activated the body is in fight or flight mode. That is a good thing at times, when it is needed. It gets our adrenalin going, like lighting a fire. But when we are constantly calling on this system it becomes overloaded, generating a chronic stress response. When the body is in constant stress mode it takes a hefty toll on our health. This ongoing chronic stress may manifest in the form of physical ailments such as inflammation, auto-immune issues, or HPA axis dysfunction, just to name a few, but the list goes on and on. This means the body is in constant tension mode and does not have the ability to refuel and heal itself. When this is the case changes need to be made, but let's not make this another source of stress for you. Baby steps my friend... you will get there.

Stress Perception

How we perceive stress is different for everyone. What I consider stressful you may think is a breeze and when your friend hears what you have on your plate, she may think she could handle that with no problem at all. The point is that we all have our own gauge as to what is stressful, and our bodies respond based on that gauge. For example, if your mother in law comes for a visit and you perceive time with her as being stressful, then you better believe your body will initiate the stress response and everything that goes with it when she shows up. I bring this up because if we can somehow change our perceptions of what is stressful, it can go a long way toward invoking that parasympathetic nervous system we spoke about earlier. For a lasting effect, we need to utilize our Parasympathetic Nervous System on a daily basis.

I took a huge step in reducing my stress level when I left a very stressful job. I know this is not an option for everyone so I am not suggesting that you go out and quit your job. What I am suggesting is that you evaluate your life. Look at the whole picture. What do you consider to be a source of stress or anxiety for you? Where and when do you feel the most anxious or agitated? Is there a way you can reframe the stressful situation or try to look at it from a different perspective? Can you look at any aspect of the stressful event and feel gratitude? I know that sounds crazy but we fall into patterns of behavior. If we can break some of these patterns, we can cut out some of the stressors in our lives.

Consider this example: A co-worker is constantly trying to take credit for your work to make herself look good in front of the boss. You work hard and this makes you furious. Instead of getting all worked up, try reframing the situation. Think of this co-worker as someone you feel sorry for as she is not creative enough to come up with her own ideas. Embrace a sense of gratitude for your own abilities and the fact that you hold yourself to a higher standard; you are ethical and have the talent to do your job well.

This is not to say that you should be a doormat either. Bottling up thoughts and feelings can also be a source of stress. For me personally, in a scenario like this, I would have to make sure the boss knows what work came from me. I would also probably throw in a statement to my co-worker like, "Wow it must feel awful, not being able to come up with your own ideas and having to swipe mine. I feel very fortunate that I have the talent and integrity to create my own work." In this example, eventually, you will no longer perceive your co-worker taking credit as stressful because you have advocated for yourself and you changed your view of this co-worker. She is no longer a threat; she is someone to be pitied, and you are calm.

Changing our perception is not easy but it is well worth the effort. In some cases, it may be as simple as repeating the change over and over to yourself or even out loud. In other cases, it may require changing your reaction to a situation. This may need to be planned out ahead of time. Even if it is scripted it still has merit as you may notice that you feel calmer afterwards. Sometimes in order to change perceptions formal treatment such as cognitive-behavioral therapy or recognizance repatterning may be warranted.

People, Places & Things

It's easy for me to tell you to reduce your stress but I get that it's not always so easy to do. First and foremost, sit and think. Really examine what aspects of your life are causing you stress as well as those that bring you joy. Look at the whole picture. Where and when do you feel the most anxious? What brings you the most pleasure or peace? How can you find more of a balance? Realistically, you may not be able to make a huge lifestyle change immediately, but small steps can lead to big sustainable change. Concentrate on your core. What I mean by this is on your purpose, relationships, and spirituality. Just like any twelve-step program says, to make real changes we must examine the people, places and things in our life.

People

Are there people in your life that are a source of negativity? These may be people you want to avoid if at all possible. The idea is to bring positive interactions and feelings your way. If there are people in your life that cause you constant stress but it is not someone that you can walk away from, then you must find ways of responding to those people that will lessen the negative effects they have on you. I will give you a personal example.

My relationship with my mother has always been toxic. While I had always hoped for better, it wasn't until I learned about the physiological effects of stress that I realized how much damage this relationship had caused me. Acceptance is a big part of reducing your stress. Coming to terms with not being able to change a situation and accepting it for what it is, is half the battle. For me, that was understanding that because of my mother's mental illness she didn't have the capacity to be the mother I wanted her to be. Okay, like I just said, accepting that fact was half the battle but dealing with her combative behavior was another story. I wish I could say I have found a way to completely eliminate the stress that is caused by this relationship, but that would not be the truth. What I have done is taken steps to find better ways of responding to her and sometimes this means putting more distance between us. I have also found some techniques to help both of us relax. Keep this in mind, as it may be helpful to share some of the relaxation techniques with others in your life. If they also utilize relaxation techniques it will make for more pleasant interactions all around. I recently found that music is a great tool for my mother. Not rocket science, right? Of course, music puts you in a good mood. But it can also be used as a therapeutic tool to reduce stress and anxiety.

Places & Situations

Are there activities or situations in your life that cause you tension? Can they be eliminated or altered in some way to be less stressful? For example, if you are heading a project at work maybe you can do some delegating so that all the tasks don't fall on you. This same principle can be applied at home. If you are planning a big holiday dinner ask that everyone bring a dish. This way you can focus on one or two dishes instead of trying to make ten different dishes yourself. Instead of doing all the house cleaning, ask your spouse and children to pitch in. If everyone does one small task it will lessen the burden you usually carry and allow you some, (dare I say it) 'free time" to unwind.

Things

Look around you. Is there something you don't like about your environment? While you may not be able to make structural changes to your home, office or yard, there are some simple changes you can make that may enhance your mood. Removing clutter and organizing your stuff can help you feel calm. When we know where things are and what we need is easily accessible, our days tend to run smoother. One way to do this is to designate areas for items. Maybe each child can have his or her own cubby or space to store their school things or sports equipment.

Color can bring life in to change the way you see your environment. Paint the room or just add something colorful to the room. Adding an accent that has a splash of color to a room can be a mood enhancer. Plants are another way to brighten up a room. They also improve air quality, which can translate into breathing better and feeling better. Check out the NASA study on house plants that improve air quality.

How about your activities? Are there activities that you enjoy doing but don't do anymore because you have too much going on with the kids, or you don't have the time because of work or other obligations? Again, it's easy for me to say 'make the time, dammit.' Take a pass on something else and make time to do something for yourself. This is important enough that I've devoted a whole chapter to it so we will dive deeper into it later.

Stressbusters

Obviously, if there is something stressful you can change or eliminate, that's a no brainer. The ideal is to avoid situations that cause you repetitive stress but since this is not always an option, we need to find positive ways to respond to them and also positive outlets for the accumulated stress. Let's look at a few simple steps you can take to invoke the relaxation response or the parasympathetic nervous system and reduce your overall stress.

Drink Water

Drinking water cleanses the toxins from your system.

Laugh

Did you ever hear the saying "Laughter is the best medicine?" Laughter actually helps to regulate the stress hormones, cortisol, and epinephrine and that will help you get your parasympathetic nervous system going. [1]

Self-Care

Take part in some type of self-care or restorative practice to invoke the parasympathetic nervous system. Examples of these practices include

Meditation, Yoga, Tai Chi, Qigong, massage, and breathwork.

Meditation

Meditation is a great way to decompress, however, many people find it difficult to do lengthy meditations, especially at first. If you can do a long meditation that is fantastic, but if you feel it isn't for you just try a short one. Even a few minutes a day can translate into big changes in the way you feel. There are several phone apps that offer quick five-to-ten-minute meditations. I have used *Headspace*, and *Breethe and Calm*. They are great because you can do it anywhere that you can get a few minutes of quiet. Eventually, you may find yourself enjoying meditation and wanting it to last longer.

Breathwork

Breathwork is another great way to reduce stress. For the most part, unless we are consciously choosing to do otherwise, we take short shallow breaths. When we concentrate on taking deep breaths (diaphragmatic breathing) we essentially communicate to the cells in our body that we are safe and all is well in the world. This allows us to enter the Parasympathetic Nervous System where the body repairs itself.

A simple way to do this is to inhale deeply and exhale thoroughly. If you can see your belly rise when you inhale you are utilizing your diaphragm. When you exhale, concentrate on pushing all the air out of the lungs. This is diaphragmatic breathing. The great thing about breathwork is that you own it. It is a simple, yet powerful tool to have in your arsenal wherever you go. You can literally do it any time you want and it works great.

Eliminate or drastically reduce your intake of processed foods.

Removing chemicals from your body will make it so your body doesn't have to work so hard to figure what these strange substances are and in turn, can relax and do the jobs it is intended to do. Elimination is ideal, but if you start by just getting the chemicals out of your diet then you are well on your way to clean eating.

Get a good night's sleep.

Good sleep is essential! Please, no technology before bed. When you look at a screen your brain thinks it is daytime and therefore does not get into the deep sleep you need to repair the damage done during the day.

Reduce caffeine

Consuming too much caffeine can also keep that Sympathetic Nervous System going as it results in the release of adrenalin. It can also affect the quality of your sleep if you have it too close to bedtime.

Exercise

Do some form of exercise. This can be a simple as a brisk walk or dancing to a song you like in your living room. This serves as a release for your stress and it works wonders for mood! Do not exercise right before going to bed as this can keep you awake.

Find quiet time

Humans need time unplugged. This is how we reboot our system. We lead busy lives with very little downtime. We are constantly experiencing information overload as we try to process everything being thrown at us. It is crucial to find some time to just be. To just be without voices or electronics or print or stimuli of any kind. In order to have peace in our lives, we need to connect with our inner selves.

A great way to do this is to connect with nature. Spend some time sitting on the beach staring at the ocean waves or taking in the beauty of the scenery in a local park, or even just going outside at night to look at the moon. Just take it in, no special thoughts and no judgment.... just be.

Connections

Nurture your relationships. This means slowing down a bit and taking the time to sit and talk or make a point of having dinner together or any other activity that gives you the chance to connect. Touch is also an important part of connecting to other humans. A hug, kiss or even holding a hand can have an instant calming effect.

Spirituality

When we feel connected to a higher power we tend to be more at ease. This can mean different things to different people. Whether you practice a religion or just do your own thing in the form of prayer, meditation or education. Regardless of what or how you practice, cultivating spirituality can translate to a sense of purpose and it is definitely a way of connecting to others. Need I say more?

A few of my favorite resources for relaxation techniques:

◊ Mindbodygreen.com
◊ Groundedmind.com

- ◊ draxe.com/stress-relievers/
- ◊ drweil.com/health-wellness/body-mind-spirit/stress-anxiety/breathing-three-exercises/
- ◊ Breethe app

Dr. Libby Weaver's book *Rushing Woman's Syndrome* is a phenomenal resource. I recommend that every woman read it, especially moms with a busy lifestyle. Dr. Weaver explains the physiological effects of not taking care of ourselves properly and offers solutions to the challenges that women face. It really is a must-read.

Nourishing You

Recently my father was hospitalized for an extended period of time. I spent a lot of time at the hospital with him and got to know some of the nurses. Let me first say that these are some of the hardest working women and men I have ever met.

On one particular day my father's nurse looked run down and I asked her if she was okay. She said she was sick. She went on to tell me how it had started as a cold but went to her chest. I said jokingly, "aren't nurses allowed to take sick days?" She said they are not supposed to take more than three sick days per year. I said how are you supposed to take care of others if you are not well? She said she feels the same way but doesn't have a choice because she has to save those three days for emergencies with her kids. I think this speaks to a failure in our way of life.

As a whole, our society does not value self-care. The notion seems to be, take some medicine and move along when the truth is that rest is what is needed to heal and rejuvenate. Health care institutions should set the precedent for how we take care of our health. I mean it is right in its name, 'health care,' right? When a health care institution is not promoting self-care, this is a systemic failure of epic proportions. When a nurse can't take a sick day or even give herself a few minutes out of her twelve-hour shift to sit down and have a cup of soup that is a problem. We are not machines and we should not be treated like machines.

We have established that more often than not we are motivated by the needs of others. We tend to be more accountable to these outside sources than we are to our own needs. There is one need of our own we seem to always acknowledge...our need to please others. Most women are natural nurturers and that is a wonderful thing. It brings us pleasure to care for others, but I must reiterate that without taking care of ourselves we will be without the precious resources we need to care for others.

When self-care is not woven into the fabric of our society, we need to make the necessary changes for ourselves. If we need to get creative and think outside of the box in order to find ways to nourish ourselves and promote self-care then that is what we must do. Try making a list of your priorities. Where do you fall on that list? Are you even on it? That's about to change.

Remember when you were at your best? In your mind try going back in time to when you felt strong and had a sense of clarity. What were you doing at that point in your life to take care of yourself? What were your outlets? How did you let off steam? It's time to revisit taking care of you. In this chapter, we will focus on tapping into your female power and learning to nourish ourselves. The goal is getting you feeling as vibrant as you did in years past. And if you never felt that way, well then, these techniques will open up a whole new world to you.

Sleep

Today is my husband's birthday. So being the angelic wife that I am, I woke him in the sweetest voice with a very special birthday present, if you know what I mean. Oh wait, you may be thinking of something else so let me set the stage.

At 12:39 A.M. I am awakened from a sound sleep by a barbaric noise that is all too familiar to me...Scott's snoring. I nudge him and the snoring calms but gradually continues to escalate again so I keep nudging. After a while (I try not to look at the clock because it makes me crazy to know exactly how much sleep I am missing). I eventually fall back to sleep.

At 1:25 A.M. I hear one of my children calling to me and I keep saying "What? I am here," but hear no reply. Eventually desperate to reach my needy child, I wake only to realize it was a dream and the person yelling "Mom, Mom" was actually my husband. His snoring was now penetrating my dreams masked as my children in need. Are you kidding? Now I am pissed. It takes a long time to fall back to sleep but eventually I do. Whew, I can still get a few hours of good sleep.... not!

At 3:32 A.M. Once again, the lumberjack cutting wood in my bedroom wakes me, but this time I know that I am done. I am wide-awake and there is no turning back. My heart is racing and so is my brain. I am thinking of everything imaginable from deadlines, to food, to my kid's health, to Christmas ornaments, to what made the dog puke this morning. You get the picture...I am wired! This time I do not fall back to sleep.

At 6:00 A.M. I have now been awake for the last two-and-a-half-hours and my angelic attributes have dulled just a bit, but I do my duty and bring them to the surface for my special birthday boy.

So, as I started saying earlier, I wake him with a very sweet "Happy Birthday, do you like what I got you? With a gentle stretch, still groggy and coming out of his peaceful slumber he asks with a smile, "What did you get me?" My reply is a little confusing to him, but I say, "I got you life! Surprise! Isn't it great? I put a lot of thought into it and thought, hey, this is one hell of a gift!"

He is clueless, so I begin to explain, "You see, while I was lying awake all night, yet again, desperate for sleep, but unable because of the intense turbulence in our bed, I reached for a pillow. I held it above your head and contemplated putting us both out of our misery." I explained to him that I eventually came to my senses and said to myself, how could I even think such a thought, after all, it is his birthday. So, I put the pillow down and lay there for the next two-and-a-half-hours until it was a reasonable time to get up." As I spoke, he just looked at me with a blank stare.

Keep in mind I am delirious at this point...sleep deprivation will do that to you, you know? Yes, sleep is the forgotten treasure. It is as necessary as food and water. Getting enough sound sleep can improve your health drastically. Not getting enough sleep or having interrupted sleep, especially on a regular basis, can be and usually is detrimental to one's health. For your sanity and your survival make sleep a priority.

"How do you sleep?" I ask my clients. The typical answer I get is "okay." When asked to describe their sleep I realize that what they deem 'okay' is anything but good enough. Sleep is an essential part of living. It is as vital as eating, drinking and breathing, yet it is taken for granted and often sacrificed by so many people.

As for me, well I've already mentioned the

physical and emotional mess that I was. I had made a conscious decision to make changes. I had researched and studied and changed so much in my life in the name of healing, but I, like many, had overlooked one of the most basic needs, the need for sleep.

When I was working outside my home, sleep had become a luxury. It was my reward only after getting all my daily tasks done. A typical day looked something like this…At the crack of dawn, throw in a load of laundry, walk and feed the dog, get everyone up and moving (no easy task) make breakfast, make sure everyone was dressed and had everything they needed for school, drive kids to their respective schools, race to work, come home from work, help kids with homework, go through paperwork, correspondence with schools, driving to practice or games, coaching softball, somehow preparing dinner, clean up from dinner and general house cleaning, make lunches for the next day all while fielding calls and emails from work, get the kids to bed, more laundry, check work emails one last time and finally go to bed.

Then in walks my husband all smiles and ready to go. My response is are you &%$#@*& kidding me? Don't get me wrong, he works hard too, but he has downtime where I do not. I am literally running all day and night. I am also the one getting up with whoever can't sleep or is sick. Then factor in the television in my bedroom and the fact that my husband snores like a bear. It was a recipe for disaster. So even when I got to bed, I didn't get to sleep and when I finally fell asleep, the snoring would continue to wake me up so any sleep I got was interrupted.

That is how it was, but not anymore. Learning about the effects of poor sleep was a slap in the face for me. It was an awakening of sorts...no pun intended.

So here I heeded the advice I received and made my bedroom my sanctuary. I stopped watching television in the bedroom and asked my husband to watch it downstairs instead of in the bedroom. I began to do some simple breathwork before bed. I do this when I lie down. This is nothing fancy. It takes about two minutes and works wonders.

Now my nights are different, and as a result, so are my days. I don't wake up irritated. I wake up feeling refreshed. I have much more energy during the day. I don't feel like I can barely keep my eyes open at two or three o'clock in the afternoon. My thinking is clearer, much less scattered. I have the ability to concentrate and be present. When someone is talking to me, I am listening and not drifting off.

My tips for a good night's sleep:

~Invest in a quality mattress that is comfortable

~ Make sleep a priority

~Keep your room dark

~No electronics for at least one hour before bed. If you have to use the computer or phone before bed try blue light blocking glasses. The blue light tricks your brain into thinking it is daytime. The brain responds accordingly saying let's go body it's time to get up, when it is really time for sleep.

~ Don't eat anything for at least an hour or more before hitting the sack.

~ Get hydrated earlier in the day. Limit the amount you drink before bed as you want to avoid having to get up to use the bathroom.

~ Try a quick meditation, breathing exercise or simple gratitude practice right before, or even when you get into bed.

If nothing seems to work, at the risk of being redundant, I recommend seeing a functional medicine doctor for a complete workup. Physical issues such as hormone imbalance and adrenal issues can also affect the quality and duration of your sleep.

Breathe

Stress management, who has time for that? I get it, you are overwhelmed. There are constant demands on you and your time. The good news is that there are some very simple things you can do to reduce your stress that require very little time.

First and foremost, you need a chance to breathe. I mean this both figuratively and also quite literally. You might be saying *duh… of course I breathe*. But I am suggesting you become mindful of your breathing and breathe deeply. When we are constantly on the go, we tend to take short shallow breaths. We benefit greatly when we breathe deeply. So, go ahead and try it, take a deep breath and watch your belly rise and fall. Notice your breath. Pay attention to it. Do it again. Breathe in and breathe out letting go of that which no longer serves you.

When you recognize your own breath the body and brain have no choice but to calm down. This practice will help you move from the sympathetic nervous system to the parasympathetic nervous system, where the body has the opportunity to refuel and regenerate.

Diaphragmatic breathing, also called baby breathing or belly breathing, is a tremendous tool. Did you ever watch a baby breathe? Their belly goes up and down. This is because they are breathing deep into their diaphragm. Innately our bodies know what to do, we just have to listen to them. We come into the world, instinctually knowing how to breathe the way we need to in order to nourish ourselves. This speaks to the third eye, listening to our intuition and our bodies. We have a lot more wisdom than we give ourselves credit for.

Breathwork (or controlled breathing) utilizes breathing exercises that improve one or more aspects of health and well-being. According to Dr. Zandra Palma of Parsley Health, "Studies have found that breathing practices can help reduce symptoms associated with anxiety, insomnia, post-traumatic stress disorder, depression and attention deficit disorder."[1]

Breathwork dates back to various ancient cultures. The common denominator among the cultures was the belief that tuning in to the rise and fall of one's breath can have life-changing effects.

Breathwork is also a great way to get to sleep. If

you are like me when you can't sleep, your brain is racing, thinking of all the things you have to get done, or things you are worried about. If you just breathe from your diaphragm and really notice each breath, your body will relax and you will fall asleep. This is better than any sleeping pill.

According to Dr. Andrew Weil, "Breathing exercises are a wonderfully effective way to reduce stress, regulate mood, and feel energized. One way to promote deeper breathing and better health is by exhaling completely. Try it: take a deep breath, let it out effortlessly, and then squeeze out a little more. Doing this regularly will help build up the muscles between your ribs, and your exhalations will naturally become deeper and longer. Start by practicing this exhalation exercise consciously, and eventually, it will become a healthy, unconscious habit." [2] Dr. Weil's website is a great resource for simple breathing exercises that can have an instant calming effect.

There are many types of breathing exercises. Among my favorites are 4-7-8 breathing, balance (square) breathing, and pranayama. Google to learn this method for yourself. The simple practice of taking a deep breath and exhaling completely is a huge step in the right direction.

Meditate

We as a society are in overdrive a great deal of the time. While technology is a wonderful tool it can also put a great deal of stress on our brains. Between our computers, smartphones, video games and other devices, images and information are constantly coming at us. Humans are not set up to be on 24/7.

There needs to be both physical and mental downtime. There is a place in our lives for looking and learning and thinking but there also needs to be a time and place for stillness. It is in the stillness that we can reach a state of peace and true stress relief.

We have talked about the importance of breathing. Meditation and breathwork go hand-in-hand, as meditation practice will help you hone in on your breathing. When meditation was first suggested to me two things came to mind. First, I don't have time, and second, I am a mover so I can't sit still long enough to mediate. But still, I agreed to give it a try. At first, I was fidgety and my brain was everywhere except on my body and breath. What I learned was that everyone's mind wanders at times. I learned not to be critical of myself for this. As soon as I stopped getting mad at myself for not doing better and just let it be, I started to notice a difference. I felt a sense of calm that I cannot say I had ever felt before. So, I took my short meditations up a notch because once a meditation began, I found myself wanting it to last longer. After a while, I began to reap some of the long-term benefits of meditation. I had heard that meditation could help improve one's ability to concentrate, reduce symptoms of depression, anxiety, and even pain.

Quite frankly I was a skeptic and did not expect to experience any of that, but I did. I felt better physically, had a sense of peace, was less anxious and much more accepting of myself. This last one was huge because I was my own worst critic, always feeling like I should have done this instead of that or should have done something better.

Mediation has helped me to experience a kind of 'it is what it is and I am what I am' attitude. I will still strive to improve in certain areas of my life where I can, but all in all, I am cool with who I am and what I do. This is a wonderful feeling, and oddly enough, one that I had not experienced until the age of forty-seven.

So, let's address the time factor. Even if you don't have time for a full mediation you can do a mini-version that will still offer you benefits. Here is one that I like to do. Identify the part or parts of your body where you feel your mood. If you can identify places in your body where you hold your emotions, particularly negative emotions, then you can ease the stress in those areas. We all have places in our bodies where we house a lot of our sadness, anger, or anxiety. This is not a conscious decision, it just happens. We need to bring a sense of calm to these areas. You can put the focus on a specific area at any time of day. You can even try this sitting at your desk at work or on the bleachers at your kid's game. I'm not saying to put your hands in the air and start chanting "ohm" in a public place. Just a minute or two of focus on your body and breath will be beneficial. Take a couple of deep breaths and concentrate on softening or relaxing those body parts that feel tense. No one even has to know you are doing it.

Also, think about where in your body you feel happiness or peace. Do you have a spring in your step? Maybe it is your feet. Do you feel strong with each breath, like every breath is a breath of fresh air? Then maybe you feel happiness in your lungs. Once you identify your happy place or places, set an intention to mentally nourish those places in your body on a daily basis. Think of this as putting gas in your happiness tank. Be mindful as you send positive energy to those places. Again, this can be done anywhere in a matter of minutes.

I find that I get an internal chuckle out of doing this when I am with a group of people or in a crowd and no one has a clue what I am doing. When you are laughing on the inside sometimes it comes out. Random laughing might look a little nutty but that's okay. If you feel compelled, share with those around you. And remember what laughter does for the body; even if it is not a full- belly laugh you still reap the benefits.

And don't forget the apps I mentioned, as many of them have quick five-to-ten- minute meditations. With this, you have calm in the palm of your hand. It's just another tool in your arsenal.

When I meditate it sets the tone for the rest of my day. I find that I am calmer and I take things in stride a little bit more. Meditation also makes me feel empowered. It is a mental memo to myself that I started my day doing something that is just for me and this something will help me have a better day.

Just say NO!

Not too long ago, when speaking with a friend she let me know her New Year's resolution. She even came up with a slogan. She called it 'Do Me 2019.' Catchy title I thought. It will certainly get attention:)

Jeanine said she was going to start doing things for herself, things that made her happy regardless of what people think. She spoke of how she was tired of doing everything for everyone else and not being appreciated for it. She went on to echo what many other moms I have spoken to over the years have said. They feel that all they do is give and they simply have nothing left to give. She was resentful, she was hurt, and more than anything, she was exhausted. Her position was not coming from a place of anger, it was simply one of a woman pushed to her physical and mental limit.

Let's go back to her original statement. "- I am going to start doing things for me regardless of what people think." Yes, this is a positive stance but what is wrong with this statement? The ending is the problem..."regardless of what people think." These five words speak volumes. These words are added to her basic statement because she is assuming that doing something, anything for herself is going to be viewed by others as selfish. She is not alone in feeling this way.

The fact is, that as moms we have been programmed to think it is selfish to take care of ourselves. We have been hardwired to take it all on ourselves and in many cases to feel like failures if we cannot do it all. We take care of our children, our husbands or partners, our homes, school/community commitments, our parents or extended family members, and in many cases do all of this while also working outside the home. Then there are those of us who work from home, which holds its own unique set of challenges. You are physically present in your home so the expectation is that you can do anything that needs to be done around the house, even though you need dedicated time to complete your work. Either way, it is a juggling act; it is 'system overload.' No one person should have to be responsible for so much without the opportunity to recharge and nurture themselves.

In business, a good leader knows how to delegate tasks and assignments. Successful companies utilize a team effort to achieve success. You would never see all the responsibilities fall on one person's shoulders. It would be an unrealistic expectation to think that the CEO could successfully handle all aspects of operations, marketing, accounting, human resources and all the rest of the departments. He or she would have individuals or teams under them to complete the various functions in order to prosper. Do you see where I am going with this? Moms are often expected to successfully handle all the responsibilities of their respective company: their family. We need to delegate!

There is a societal norm here that is problematic. It is the idea that we are less if we don't do it all. It is the belief that if we do not take care of everyone and everything and basically neglect ourselves, then we are not good mothers. What a load of crap!

I have to go back to the plane analogy again. When you get on a plane the flight attendant explains that in the event of an emergency it is vital you put on your own oxygen mask before helping anyone else with theirs. This is basic, people ...if we can't breathe how can we help others? Oh, and yes this is an emergency! We are losing ourselves. If we are not healthy and dare I say 'happy' how can we be expected to take care of those around us? How can we be expected to be calm and pleasant when we are stressed to our limit?

Here is the answer...It is not selfish to do things for yourself. I was Jeanine two years ago. I was on the verge of a nervous breakdown. I was like the Energizer Bunny. I just kept going and going and going without any means to recharge. I was taking care of my three kids (four if you include my husband) providing care to my aging parents, doing all the cooking, laundry, school-related activities, coaching, and I had a job that was psychologically stressful. I was in physical pain, I was moody, I was short-tempered and easily agitated. I had become someone I did not recognize.

So, what did I do? The first thing was to say NO. That's right I said 'no.' You see, I realized that almost everything was either asked or demanded of me. So, I thought to myself what would happen if I just said no? "Mom, can you get this?" No. "Mom, I need you to do this" .... No. Of course, I didn't deny them important services. I said no to the stupid things that were asked of me out of sheer laziness. For example, when my daughter is actually closer to the refrigerator than I am and says, "Mom can you get me a drink?" The answer is no. The first time something like that is asked, I do explain that at this age she is perfectly capable of getting herself a drink. After a while they get the message, which is, you are capable and I am not your servant.

When asked to commit time you really don't have to a PTA fundraiser, it is okay to say no. 'No' does not have to be followed by excuses or justification. It's okay to just say "No." There need not be guilt or shame associated with this response. Okay, if you want to be really nice, you can make it, "No Thank you."

Occasionally you may need, or just really want, to give a little more than a simple no. For example, when my husband says to me, "We need more toilet paper in our bathroom." If you can imagine with comments like this one, Raven makes an appearance. My response..."You're kidding, right? You are reporting to me that toilet paper needs to be brought from downstairs to upstairs as if this is my job? You spend so much time in the bathroom one might think it was your second job.... I think you can handle carrying your tools of the trade up a flight of stairs." So, as I said some circumstances warrant a little more than a no and occasionally my sarcasm gets the best of me, but remember 'no' is a complete sentence and there is nothing wrong with using it by itself.

When asked to take on extra responsibilities you don't have the time or desire for, it is okay to say "No." When my husband tells me something my son or daughter did wrong and then says, "Let's do something about that," meaning you deal with it, my answer is No.

So, I started saying no like crazy just for the fun of it, Mom get me this, honey I need this .... No, no, no! It is fun and very entertaining to see the look of bewilderment on their faces as if I had just shot The Queen.

The Takeaway~ We are not bad for needing time to ourselves. Everyone needs me time. If a car has no gas left it stands to reason it will not run. If your proverbial gas tank is empty it needs filling before you break down on the side of the road. Do yourself a favor and fill up with some high test 'NO'!

Have an Accountability Partner

Early in my health coaching program, we were asked to find an 'accountability partner.' We were to connect with this person every week to offer each other support and keep each other accountable for staying on task. I saw this as a major nuisance. I mean really, I am a grown woman. Did I really need a stranger making sure that I am doing what I am supposed to do? And if I need support, I have friends that I can go to. This sounded ridiculous to me!

So out of a virtual sea of students, we were asked to find someone who was a good fit for us. Again, I am annoyed. I mean really how am I supposed to do this? This is just one more thing on my To-Do list that I don't want to do or have time for. Regardless of my aversion to the process, I needed to fulfill my graduation requirements so I went on my way putting myself out there to find a fellow sucker. After a few offers that didn't feel right, I went with a woman named Lisa.

Okay progress, I could check finding someone off my list. Now I would just do my weekly phone call with Lisa and check that off my list too. In my mind, this was an obligation I just needed to fulfill, no different than an assignment or test.

But this was different. At first, Lisa and I just stuck to the program, reviewing school work and assuring each other that we were both on task. Over time we realized that although we had very different lives there were many common threads. We began to speak more freely and eventually became very comfortable with one another. We built a relationship and a real connection. The keyword being 'real.' There was no fluff involved. We say what we think and what we really feel, not what we think we should be saying or feeling. This hour a week was no longer an obligation, it was something I very much looked forward to. I enjoyed talking to Lisa and having that designated time to talk was liberating. It was therapeutic in a sense because this became a safe space for both of us. We could say anything and the other would give genuine, honest feedback without judgment. Lisa has become a huge source of support in my life and I am now proud to call her my friend.

Lisa and I both graduated and obviously are no longer required to have our weekly talks, but we still talk on a regular basis. As it turns out, this accountability partner that I didn't want to find became a trusted friend who I value more than words can say.

If someone had suggested that I take an hour a week to talk with a friend, I would have said there was no way. I simply don't have the time. But being forced to make the time as part of my school requirements was actually a blessing in disguise. I learned the true value of support. I didn't realize how much I needed it until I had it. Don't get me wrong, I have friends I could call at any time, but the truth is that we all lead busy lives and would have never made time for this.

We do the occasional girl's night out and get together with our husbands and kids, but we would have never thought to designate regular time that is just for us. Let's face it, as moms this is another 'me thing' that we don't do because we tend to put ourselves at the bottom of the list. But remember ladies, if our spouse or child needed designated time, we would make the time. We need to make the time for ourselves.

The Takeaways~

1- Get the support you need. The journey as a mom these days is tough enough, but doing it without support is crazy. Make the time for you. Reach out to a friend or even an acquaintance with the idea of being each other's accountability partner or whatever you want to call it. Regardless of your individual paths, you will support each other in your respective journeys. Set up a designated time to talk and remember that this time must be sacred. Treat it as a business meeting or an obligation to someone else, that way you will be less inclined to cancel. Another way to get the support you need is to start a small group where you all meet or talk regularly to share. I would suggest keeping the group small in order for each person to have ample floor time so to speak. You can do one-on-one or a group in whatever setting works for you, over the phone, a weekly walk, or meet at the beach or a café. Whatever works for you…get creative!

2- Things happen for a reason and we need to be open to the possibilities. Sometimes God or the powers that be put people in our lives for a reason. Although I didn't know it, I needed this person in my life. Voila, and here she is. So, when you don't see the value in something initially, take a step back and say, 'hey maybe there is a reason for this. Maybe there is a big picture, a silver lining or something larger at play.' Keep an open mind and you may be pleasantly surprised.

Find Your Tribe

In a world where we are always 'plugged in,' human interaction is more important than ever. We need to disconnect from devices and connect with people. Heard of the Blue Zones? According to Dan Buettner, these are geographic regions of the world where people live long lives and have low rates of chronic disease.[1] Although each of these regions live differently from one another they share some commonalities. Among them is their value of family, and the social network. In each of them, emphasis is placed on taking the time to connect with one's spouse, kids and parents as well as making time to be social with those around them. [1]

So how do we achieve this? I believe that it starts with finding our respective tribes. I'm sure you have heard the phrase "Find your tribe" before. But what does that really mean? Who is your tribe? Well, that is up to you. Your tribe may be your family. Your tribe may be your friends. Your tribe may be your neighbors. Your tribe may be a group of people who you share one common bond with. Your tribe may be a combination of all of these. Or your tribe may look totally different. The people that belong to your tribe is all up to you. Your tribe doesn't have to be huge. It could even be just one or two people.

What is important is that you connect with your tribe regularly and that your tribe is made up of people who accept you for who you are. They should be people you can be honest with without fear of rejection. They should be people with whom you don't have to put on airs or appear perfect. They should be people who respect and cherish their connection to you, as much as you respect and cherish your connection to them. The more real you are the more you will connect with your tribe.

Pay attention to the people around you and savor relationships. Prioritize how you relate to those in your life. If you feel like you don't have a tribe then create one. Join social groups or clubs. Reach out to connect with old friends or family that you haven't seen in a while. It can even be an online community. Although I feel like the best connections are made face-to-face. It will be worth your time and effort. So, find your tribe and make it a priority to connect with them regularly!

Cultivate Good Smells

Smell is a potent wizard that transports you across thousands of miles and all the years you have lived. ~ Helen Keller

Did you ever get a whiff of something and find yourself transported to another place and time? How do you feel when you walk into the house and immediately smell the fragrant aroma of a home-cooked meal? Our sense of smell can bring back a memory, help us to recall a feeling and even transform a mood.

As my dad used to say, "The nose knows," meaning you get a lot of information from your sense of smell. Turns out that while he didn't know it, there is some science behind this simple statement.

"Scents can have positive effects on mood, stress reduction, sleep enhancement, self-confidence, and physical and cognitive performance," says Theresa Molnar, executive director of the Sense of Smell Institute, the research and educational arm of the perfume industry's Fragrance Foundation. By becoming more aware of the way specific odors affect you personally, you may be able to enhance your health and well-being." [1]

Last year, an electrician came to my house to fix an issue we were having. He is a friend of my husband so he had been to our house before. As soon as he came in, he said "I love coming here. You are always cooking something and it always smells awesome. It puts me in such a good mood." This sent me over the moon because cooking is one of the major ways that I show love. I cook for my family and my friends. When someone is sick or hurt or sad, I cook for them. Hearing someone say that just the smell of my cooking made him feel good, made me feel incredible. It also made me realize how powerful scent can be.

According to the Social Issues Research Center, "Our olfactory receptors are directly connected to the limbic system, the most ancient and primitive part of the brain, which is thought to be the seat of emotion. Smell sensations are relayed to the cortex, where 'cognitive' recognition occurs, only after the deepest parts of our brains have been stimulated. Thus, by the time we correctly name a particular scent as, for example, 'vanilla,' the scent has already activated the limbic system, triggering more deep-seated emotional responses."[2]

A great read on this topic is The Scent of Desire by Rachel Herz, Ph.D. Dr. Herz explores the science behind our sense of smell and how it's directly linked to our health and well-being.

"Aromatherapy, also referred to as Essential Oil therapy, can be defined as the art and science of utilizing naturally-extracted aromatic essences from plants to balance, harmonize and promote the health of body, mind, and spirit. It seeks to unify physiological, psychological and spiritual processes to enhance an individual's innate healing process. [3]

Used for centuries around the world, essential oils are a great way to utilize your sense of smell to enhance your mood and health. Essential oils can be used alone or in combination with other oils. Some brands make blends created specifically for calming purposes. You can even purchase jewelry that releases small amounts of essential oils or mini diffusers for your car. All oils are not created equal, so it is important to buy from a reputable source. Real essential oils are potent so do your homework before using to determine the proper usage and method. For example, some oils, when applied topically, require a carrier oil for dilution and/or proper absorption. It is also important to note that some oils are not safe for use during pregnancy, while nursing or on infants.[4]

One of my favorite resources for essential oil use is Smart Mom's Guide to Essential Oils by Dr.

Maria Snyder. Dr. Snyder gives information on how to choose and use essential oils as well as a ton of great recipes for everything from diffuser or topical blends to cleaning and personal care products. Another great resource is Dr. Josh Axe's website: draxe.com/section/natural-remedies/essential-oils/. He has a ton of information on all things essential oils.

If there is a particular smell that resonates with you, then make smelling it a priority. For example, I absolutely love the smell of lemongrass so I use it frequently. There are many scents that can be helpful in reducing stress and anxiety.[5] Luckily for me, lemongrass happens to be one of them. I can absolutely say that this scent has a positive effect on me it has become my 'go-to' scent when I am feeling stressed out.

There are plenty of opportunities to utilize your sense of smell as a way to enhance your well-being without spending a dime. Sniff in to smell the awesome aroma of the orange you are about to eat. But wait, it doesn't end there. Don't throw that peel away. Instead, put it in a small pot with some water and a few drops of vanilla extract and simmer for a few minutes. Your whole house will soon be filled with the aromatic scent of citrus and vanilla which can both be used as mood enhancers.

A word of caution...it is important that good smells come from good things. Some commercial products that smell good may contain chemicals that are toxic. These products include some air fresheners, candles, room sprays, and cleaning products. The same holds true for many lotions, body sprays, perfumes, and personal hygiene products. Whenever possible, opt for products with ingredients that are botanically based and do not contain a laundry list of chemicals.

Our sense of smell is powerful. I believe the more you use your third eye and tap into that mind-body connection, the more powerful this sense will become. So, I mean it quite literally when I say take the time to smell the roses. Next time you step outside, take a deep breath. Take a moment to notice what you smell. Each season offers a different scent and feeling. Take in the smell of the ocean when you are at the beach. Smell the crisp fall air. Or try one of my daughters' favorite things, sitting on a rocking chair on the porch and smelling the beautiful scent of the summer rain. Close your eyes and savor the smell of an apple pie baking in the oven. The possibilities are endless. All you have to do is take the time to notice them. So, go ahead and surround yourself with smells you love!

Dance

Did you ever see a sign that says dance like no one's watching? Well, whoever came up with that phrase is a genius. Dancing is a great release. Not only is it a great release of anxiety and frustration, but it is exercise too. Dancing is also a creative outlet. So, if you are like me and feel like you don't have a creative bone in your body, start dancing and you might be surprised to find out that you do. Just like singing, go crazy when you dance. Don't even think about the moves, just let your body feel the music and start moving to it. I don't care if you dance like Elaine from *Seinfeld*, just let it fly.

Don't have time? Do it while you are doing something else. As silly as this sounds it is a fun way to get things done. I like to 'dance clean.' I dance while I am cleaning the house. I put my headphones on, crank up my favorite music and away I go. Or sometimes I skip the headphones and blast the music throughout the house. Either way, I am getting my heart rate up, releasing endorphins and my house has never looked better. If someone was watching, would they think I was a little nuts? Absolutely, but that is okay. I feel great during and after my dance-cleaning. This is nourishing me and it can nourish you too.

Daydream

Let yourself go there! Where? That's totally up to you. Maybe it is to a great memory with an old boyfriend or girlfriend. Maybe it is someone or something that you fantasize about. It doesn't even have to be real. You can create a fantasy in your head. Either way, you need to go to a time and place where you are a rock star. In this place you may be experiencing attraction, pleasure, excitement, joy, passion or power, either individually or, if it all at once, kudos to you.

Daydreaming brings you to another time and place, which can do wonders for your mood. It's okay to daydream about a scenario that you would like to happen or even an event from your past. The key is to daydream about something or someone that brings about positive feelings.

Maybe your ego needs a boost, so go back in your mind to a time when you looked your best and got a little more attention than you do now. A good throwback song can help get you there too. Maybe it is that boyfriend or girlfriend from your past that elicited feelings you want to feel again. But it doesn't have to be something from the past. This is your show...it can be something you envision in the future or something you wish would happen or even some characters you make up and bring to life in your mind. You set the stage and away you go. Just remember the important thing is that this should make you feel awesome. If you find yourself going to a place that makes you sad, angry or uneasy in any way then switch gears and find a new fantasy.

Some people may feel like this is being disloyal to your partner. I say no way! You have a right to your own thoughts and feelings and you have a need to feel good about yourself. And let's not kid ourselves, everyone fantasizes, including our spouses. Oh, and let's not forget that men make no apologies for doing this, so neither should we. This is your fantasy or daydream and whether or not you want to share it with your partner is completely up to you. Some of mine I share and others I keep to myself, but either way, my husband definitely benefits from this practice because daydreaming lights a spark in me. Given the chance, it could do the same for you. Sharing fantasies with each other may even bring new life and excitement to your relationship. Allowing yourself the freedom to go there (wherever your 'there' is) without reservation and without guilt is freeing. Don't be surprised if this practice sparks creativity within you and even with your partner, essentially making you a better partner in the long run. Ladies, it is the least you can do for your husbands;)

Sweat

Are there occasions when you feel like you want to scream or hit something? Lots of people take meds to stop feeling this way. Before turning to the medicine cabinet try a bout of exercise. You don't have to turn into a fitness guru but a little exercise each day or even a couple of times a week goes a long way toward relieving stress and increasing energy.

According to studies at Harvard University, "The mental benefits of aerobic exercise have a neurochemical basis. Exercise reduces levels of the body's stress hormones, such as adrenaline and cortisol. It also stimulates the production of endorphins, chemicals in the brain that are the body's natural painkillers and mood elevators. " [1]

Additionally, sweating is one of the best ways to eliminate toxins such as Phthalates, BPA and heavy metals from the body. [2]

When, at age forty-five, I learned that I was at the beginning stage of osteoporosis (another result of poor nutrition in my youth) my doctor recommended weight training. She explained that it was important for me to build my bones before entering menopause and that this was a great way to do it. Lift weights? Really? Wasn't there another way I thought? Ugh, this was the last thing I wanted to do. But like it or not, this was what I needed. Knowing I only had a small window of opportunity before my body began these changes, I followed her advice. After all, if I didn't address this now this was sure to lead to major issues down the road.

In order to learn proper techniques and avoid injury, I decided to work with a personal trainer. Even though this was an added expense that definitely wasn't in the budget, I saw it as an investment in myself so I found a way to do it. I did my research and got a trainer that listened to my needs and tailored a program that would work for me. If you decide to go this route, I recommend doing your homework first and don't feel that you have to sign on with a trainer or gym that you are not comfortable with. I am grateful I was able to find an incredible trainer who has supported me in my quest for better health. She has provided me with a great deal of education with respect to technique, which will continue to serve me down the road when I am training on my own. My trainer also helped me become more in tune with my body's strengths and weaknesses and more importantly how to make the necessary adjustments.

There is one more aspect of this training that I must mention. I love it. I absolutely love weight training. I expected not to like it. I expected it to be a chore, one more thing on my huge To-Do list, but it isn't. It's the funniest thing when you think you know what you will like or not like and you end up being totally wrong. It makes it all that much better. I look forward to my training sessions and I dread having to miss one. After weight training, I feel more energetic and calmer all at the same time. I feel strong and I feel proud of myself for what I accomplish and for remaining true to myself. And did I mention that I feel strong? Yes, of course, I am getting physically stronger but I also feel stronger mentally. It is an amazing feeling!

I am not telling you to go out and start lifting weights. This is what works for me but everyone is different. I tell you this story because just like me, I know that many of you are reluctant to add in the exercise. My point here is that if you just give exercise a try you may end up loving it. It doesn't have to be weight training or running or anything strenuous. Everyone is different so it is important to find an exercise regimen that works for you. Consult your physician to determine the best course for you. Even just a brisk walk will get that heart rate up, which will get those endorphins going. Exercise is a total stress buster!

Massage

I'm sure I don't have to tell you that massage is a great stress reliever. We would all love a regular massage but let's face it most of us don't have the time or the disposable income. I have the perfect solution…it is free, you can do it as often as you like and it is right in our own home.

Yes, you guessed it, it's your very own showerhead! Take it from me, this everyday device can work wonders! If you don't already have one, please do yourself a favor and invest in a unit with a hand-held piece that you can adjust for different effects. Believe me, it is worth it.

Follow my lead. Close your eyes, imagine you are on a tropical island (or any place that makes you happy). For the purposes of this example, we will go with the tropical island. You can be alone or with the companion or your choice. Remember, it is your happy place, your private happy place, so it can be wherever you want with whoever you want. Ready, let's begin. Close your eyes, hear the waves breaking on the shore, feel the cool ocean breeze on your skin. The smell of coconut is all around you. Now that we have set the stage, envision you are receiving the best massage you have ever had. Use the pulsating shower massage any place you feel tension in your body (or even places that you don't;). Use your imagination and get the most out of it. Before you know it, you will find that you are feeling very relaxed, your muscles are not so achy and the best part, you get a few minutes or maybe even a half-hour, depending on how big your hot water tank is, of PEACE!

Get creative with this, ladies. You can soothe sore muscles or use the shower massage to bring you extra pleasure. Okay, so I lied, it's not totally free…you may find yourself enjoying the water massage so much that your frequency and duration causes an increase in your water bill. Well worth it, I say!

Tip: Make sure to tell your spouse and kids that you need some privacy so you can get the full effect without, the "Mom I need…." bringing the relaxation to a screeching halt.

Laugh

"A day without laughter is a day wasted."~ Charlie Chaplin

Growing up with a mom who suffered from severe anxiety was, well, let's just say tension was a way of life for me. My dad was not an educated man, yet he was more in tune with the balance of things than most people. He was a joker. Comic relief was his forte. He could turn any situation into something to laugh about. Whether it was telling a joke, speaking in his made-up language or randomly bursting into song, he made me laugh. There were times when this drove me nuts as it was hard to even get a straight answer out of the man without him slipping some type of pun into the mix. As I got older, I realized that my dad's humor was an amazing gift in my life. He laughed at himself and in doing so taught me to laugh at myself.

At age eighty-eight my father accompanied me when taking my mother to the neurologist. He was in pretty bad physical shape himself at this point and some would say he didn't have a lot to laugh about.

Throughout the visit, he cracked one joke after another. He said, "Doc my wife is a great driver, in fact, she was rated the second-best driver in the whole state of New Jersey." With a look of bewilderment, the doctor asked "Really?" "Oh yes, it's true," he said. Then he followed with, "Everyone else in the state tied for first." The doctor seemed to be annoyed by his antics. She scolded him in a way, saying, "This is very serious. It is not funny. Do you make jokes about everything?" He looked at her kind of puzzled and replied, " Well yes, yes I do. If you can't laugh at life then what is the point?" She just shook her head at him. A few moments passed and he said, "I like you. You are a good doctor. You need to laugh a little though." I thought for sure she would ask him to leave the exam room, but she didn't. Funny thing was, as we were getting ready to leave her office, the doc pulled me aside and said, "He is adorable, make sure you bring him to your mother's next visit."

That is the way my father has lived his life, making people smile and laugh. He has given me this gift of comedy which has alleviated incredible stressors in my life. I believe that along with my faith, what kept me sane was the fact that he made me laugh daily and for this, I am eternally grateful.

The bottom line is that laughter can incite a whole host of positive physiological effects on your body. The chronic stress response that we discussed earlier can be stopped in its tracks with our body's 'feel-good' hormones that are released when we laugh. When you are not in a pattern of chronic stress the body's immune system works more efficiently. Simply put, when you laugh, tension is released, positive thoughts are formed and you work a few muscles in the process without even hitting a gym. Sounds like a home run to me. But don't take my word for it. Let's look at the science behind this concept.

Dr. Lee Berk of Loma Linda University and his colleagues have studied the effects of laughter on the human body. They discovered a connection between laughter and the production of anti-bodies and endorphins (the body's natural pain killers). They also found that laughter helps to regulate the stress hormones, cortisol, and epinephrine. [1]

According to health and wellness educators at the Chopra Center, there's a contraction of muscles when you laugh that increases blood flow and oxygenation, stimulating the heart and lungs and triggering the release of endorphins that help you feel more relaxed both physically and emotionally. [3]

So maybe you feel like you don't have a lot to laugh about right now. That is the whole point. You need to find something that will make you laugh. It can be tuning in to a sitcom that you find funny, listening to a comedy station in your car, or my personal favorite is getting together with friends with whom you are able to let loose and laugh with. There is even laughter therapy and laughter yoga if you need a little help getting your funny on. So, get started and tickle that funny bone!

Sing Like You're a Rock Star

This is a stress reliever you can do anywhere. Sing. No, don't just sing, sing at the top of your lungs. That's right, reach way down deep, use that diaphragm and belt it out.

Okay so you may not feel comfortable doing this at work or in the grocery store but I assure you if you find a place to do it, you will keep doing it. I used to only sing when I was alone, usually in my car, but now I belt one out in front of my kids or husband or wherever. The kids have been mortified when I have gone so far as to sing or dance in a public place but that is okay. Do they think I am nuts? Absolutely! But I would rather them see me being whacky or silly then being angry because of pent up frustration or unreleased stress.

When the situation warrants quick comic relief there is nothing better than belting out a tune. I even ask my kids to sing along but I usually just get strange looks or laughter. You may be thinking, how does having my kids laugh at me help the situation. Trust me, laughter helps all situations.

While singing with or in front of others is great, I feel that I personally get the maximum benefit when I am alone. Driving in my car is my favorite spot. It must be the acoustics because I feel like a rock star in my car. Let loose, just don't forget to keep your hands on the wheel and eyes on the road if your concert takes place while driving.

I find the music that speaks to me and I belt out the tunes. That's right I sing at the top of my lungs like I am Whitney, Adele or Rhianna. If I'm in a country mood then lookout Carrie and Miranda cause here I come. You may be the worst singer ever, maybe even completely tone-deaf (God knows I am) but not in this space. Here you're a card-carrying, autograph-signing, 'can't make it to PTA on Tuesday because I am on tour this week,' rock star! Try it.

Singing loud and strong releases tension like you can't even imagine. You use your diaphragm so it is right in line with belly breathing. Singing works for all moods. It enhances a good mood and usually improves a bad mood. Sad today? Belt out a really sad song about someone who has been wronged or maybe a happy, upbeat song will do the trick. This depends on your needs. Once you find what works for you, run with it. It is as good as an hour in a therapist's chair without the copay. If you are angry, you get out your anger without unleashing an irrational tirade on another human. FYI: Raven loves to sing!

As I said, alone is great but there is also a perk to doing this in front of others or even with others. People may laugh at you, with you, look at you like you are crazy or maybe all of the above. Either way, when this happens, you can't help but laugh at yourself. For me there is no choice in the matter, it makes me crack up. Laughing at yourself is so beneficial. It is humbling, and relaxing, and remember those endorphins (happy hormones) released with laughter.

Tip: Have your favorite music on hand when you know you are going to need a rock star moment. I have different songs for my different moods. I find that singing along to a strong female voice can be especially empowering.

O Yes!

The last topic that I am going to talk about in the *Nourishing You* chapter is sexual health and in particular, orgasm. That's right I said it, Orgasm! I know traditionally this topic is taboo, especially for women, but it is important, so here goes. Like men, women need to have orgasms. It is a way to help yourself feel good both physically and mentally.

According to researchers at the Mayo Clinic, "Women's sexual health, like men's, is important to overall emotional and physical well-being."

They go on to say that "A fulfilling sex life improves your sleep quality and reduces stress. [1]

Orgasm reduces stress hormones and anxiety, relieves headaches and helps you get a good night's sleep. It also helps increase your DHEA (an anti-aging hormone) that improves your brain health, the appearance of your skin, and your immune function. It can also act as a natural anti-depressant and help improve your mood.[2]

So we have established that sex is beneficial but I get that it is not always a priority when you are exhausted and overwhelmed, and especially if you feel like it is one more thing being asked of you by someone else. Believe me, I understand this feeling. If this is how it feels for you then go back to the science here and remind yourself of the health benefits it will bring to you. This is really a win/win. Obviously, your partner will be thrilled if things amp up in this department, but so will you. You can have all the physiological and psychological benefits described above.

Listen, the bottom line is that getting where you need to get with your partner is awesome, but if for whatever reason that is not working for you then it is not necessary. No, I am not suggesting that you cheat on your spouse or partner. Quite the contrary. I am suggesting that you open the lines of communication. For example, if your partner needs a little help with technique to get you there then I suggest an open dialogue to address this. You don't necessarily need expert advice. You are the expert on you and who knows your body better than you? You can be the tour guide. You can also ask him if he might like something done differently. Or maybe the two of you might want to try something new. The important thing is to communicate. It might be a little awkward at first but once you call out the elephant in the room, great things can happen.

Regardless of what your sex life with your partner looks like, you can also take care of business on your own, if you know what I mean. As science suggests, the benefits of orgasm are enormous. So, make time for yourself and make this a priority. As my Qigong master says "Self-love is self-care." So, go ahead and take care of yourself today. You will be glad you did!

Side note: This is yet another reason that making sure your hormones are in balance. Your hormones affect your sex drive, so get them checked!

Nutrition

"Let food be the medicine and medicine be the food," ~ Hippocrates

Food for Pleasure & Power

The way you eat has a lot to do with the way you digest and absorb the nutrients in your food. Food should bring you pleasure. It should be experienced and savored. Eating this way puts us in a relaxed state, bringing peace to our bodies and minds, which helps us to better digest our food. When we are rushing and stressed out, we tend to not chew our food completely or as well as we should. The more we chew our food the better it is for our digestion and absorption of nutrients. Taking the time to savor a meal with family and friends also enhances our social connections.

If you can change the way you think about food it can be life-changing. In addition to thinking of food as something to be enjoyed, try thinking of food as fuel for your body. This fuel translates to power. If you can envision that everything you put into your mouth is a different type of fuel, even better. So, candy, cake or a high-sugar-processed snack will give you a quick boost but it will be followed by a crash. Is that what you need to get you through your day? Now think of the alternative. If you put a whole food such as a fruit or vegetable into your body you are giving your body the high test. It is going to take care of you for the long haul.

If you're craving carbs, have carbs, but opt for one that will serve you well. For example, if you eat a Big Mac you will get your carbs but you will get the simple carbs that only offer you a quick fix along with pseudo meat, trans fats, and additives. Let's check out the carb component of this meal ...the Big mac bun:

Ingredients: *Enriched Flour (Bleached Wheat Flour, Malted Barley Flour, Niacin, Reduced Iron, Thiamin Mononitrate, Riboflavin, Folic Acid), Water, High Fructose Corn Syrup and/or Sugar, Yeast, Soybean Oil and/or Canola Oil, Contains 2% or Less: Salt, Wheat Gluten, Calcium Sulfate, Calcium Carbonate, Ammonium Sulfate, Ammonium Chloride, Dough Conditioners (May Contain One or More of: Sodium Stearoyl Lactylate, DATEM, Ascorbic Acid, Azodicarbonamide, Mono and Diglycerides, Ethoxylated Monoglycerides, Monocalcium Phosphate, Enzymes, Guar Gum, Calcium Peroxide), Sorbic Acid, Calcium Propionate and/or Sodium Propionate (Preservatives), Soy Lecithin, Sesame Seed.* [1]

That doesn't even touch on the junk found in the rest of the meal. Then there is the cheese and sauce with laundry lists of ingredients that look much like that of the bun. Okay, well at least the meat is good, right? Is it grass-fed beef, free of hormones and antibiotics? I don't think so. There is nothing here that is going to give you any serious fuel for your body. Quite the contrary. Your body will use its precious energy trying to digest these ingredients that it doesn't recognize. Your body will be screaming inside…hell no!

On the flip side, if you eat a bowl of quinoa or brown rice with arugula, seasoned simply with olive oil, lime & sea salt you get your carbs along with some healthy fat, vitamins and minerals. Your body will say Yes, I can use this!

So, what I am suggesting is that you actually think about the positive (or negative) effects of what you are putting in your body. I like to envision Popeye eating his spinach. This may sound silly but visualization like this can really help change your mindset. Before you know it, instead of craving sweets you may start craving fruits or veggies. By adding in more whole foods you are essentially crowding out the bad stuff. If you try this there will not be much room left for the bad stuff. This may even translate into eliminating a lot of junk food long term. You may start to feel the need to get a good amount of whole foods or efficient fuel into your body before adding in any sweets.

If you were assembling a multidisciplinary team at work, when looking at possible candidates, you would ask what does this person bring to the table. Think of what you eat in the same way. You need all the bases covered because you are using food for fuel, so ask yourself "What does this food bring to the table." No pun intended, but seriously look at that food and say, "What can you do for me?"

This can be (in a general sense) to achieve overall well-being, or it can be more specific depending on what is going on with your body. In other words, you can use foods to aid with a specific issue. For example, if I am nursing an injury I would turn to food with anti-inflammatory properties, such as turmeric, wild-caught salmon, shiitake mushrooms, green tea, papaya, blueberries, extra virgin olive oil, broccoli, kelp, sweet potato and hot peppers such as cayenne or chili pepper. If I am going to be flying on an airplane, I am going to want to promote blood flow and reduce the effects of radiation which can be accomplished with greens, sea vegetables, chlorella, spirulina or mushrooms.

What is it that you need right now? Do your

homework and grab your fork!

Grandma's Rolling

Before I knew anything about nutrition, I would find myself saying "My grandmother would be rolling over in her grave if she saw this." I was referring to what I was eating, specifically the processed foods I was serving to my family. So even though I had no formal nutrition education at the time, on some deeper level I knew there was something very wrong with this picture. I am not claiming to be clairvoyant here. What I am saying is that we all know this intuitively, but many of us have lost our way.

Let me be clear that losing our way is through no fault of our own. In a sense, we have been brainwashed by advertising. We are bombarded with messages about what we should eat and most of these messages are driven by deep pockets rather than common sense. Who sends these messages? Food companies. Who allows this to happen? Uncle Sam.

The resistance of many of the major food companies to label GMOs is evidence of their motivation. This seems simple enough, right? We should know what we are eating. Sixty-four countries around the world require the labeling of genetically modified foods. Since the United

States is ahead of the curve in most areas, it seems like a no-brainer that the US would label GMOs, right? Wrong! Unlike most other developed countries – such as twenty-eight nations in the European Union, Japan, Australia, Brazil, Russia, and even China, the U.S. has no laws requiring labeling of genetically modified food.[1] Finally, that was changed but companies still have two years before that have to comply. On January 1, 2020 a national mandatory bioengineered (BE) food disclosure standard (NBFDS or Standard) was implemented. The new Standard requires food manufacturers, importers, and other entities that label foods for retail sale to disclose information about BE food and BE food ingredients. This was long overdue and mandatory compliance is still not until January 1, 2022.[2]

I know what you are thinking, that doesn't make any sense. And you're right. It doesn't make sense to us, the consumers, because we make choices based on what will benefit us. But the motivation of many of the major food companies is quite different. Plain and simple, labeling GMOs will cost them money. Their bottom line is always money, which has nothing to do with the health of the people consuming their product.

There is a whole realm of food politics that many

people are completely unaware of, yet these lobbies influence our daily lives in a huge way. Have you heard of Big Pharma? Well, there is Big Food too. The big food conglomerates have very deep pockets, which they use to influence the information that is funneled to the public.

For example, we have all heard the slogan "Milk. It does a body good." Millions of dollars each year are spent by the dairy industry to push this message. But does it? Does milk really do a body good? Maybe, but maybe not. There is certainly substantial information suggesting that milk does not do a body good. We now know that it is directly linked to inflammation. This inflammation can manifest in different ways for different people, such as autoimmune disease, digestive issues, and acne, just to name a few. Yet with all this information out there, dairy has remained a part of the USDA's Food Pyramid, now known as 'My Plate,' with no statement to warn that dairy may not be a good choice for everyone. They list it as one of the five food groups, essential to getting the nutrients that you need. Why do you think that is? Sure, calcium and Vitamin D are important but there are plenty of whole food sources for those nutrients. You don't need milk to get them. Why doesn't the USDA point that out?

Two reasons...

1 - The deep pockets that I referred to in the paragraphs above have reached our government in the form of lobbyists who persuade Congress in a huge way.

2- The government subsidizes certain food industries, such as meat, sugar, dairy, corn, and wheat.

As a result of government subsidies, prices for fruits and vegetables can seem high in comparison to the products receiving the subsidies. In other words, produce is pricey for a reason. I've gotten a little off the beaten path here, but this is a topic that is near and dear to my heart. It is important for all Americans to be aware that there are choices being made for us and these choices are not always in our best interest. We cannot blindly trust that the food on the shelves at our local grocery store is good for us, even if the FDA or USDA says it is. In some cases, even calling it *food* is a stretch when you look at all the preservatives, chemicals, and additives contained in it.

The bottom line is that it is up to us to educate ourselves, read labels, ask questions and take a stand. Taking a stand can mean different things to different people. It can mean lobbying against

Big Food or it can be as simple as spreading the word and choosing not to buy products made by companies that do not put the public's best interest first. The point is that we need to send a collective message that we want the whole truth and will accept nothing less.

All Roads Lead to Your Gut

There are a lot of things you can do to help yourself but among the greatest is to take processed, chemicalized, "pseudo" foods out of your diet. Our bodies do not recognize these man-made chemicals and synthetics as food. Why? Because they are not food. Our bodies are really amazing, well-oiled machines that carry out so many functions instinctually but digesting these alien substances is not one of them. But because it is so intelligent your body will make the necessary adjustments to accommodate the presence of these foreign species. Unfortunately, the adjustments it needs to make can cause you significant harm in the long run.

Because the body doesn't recognize these foreign substances, it can see them as invaders and attack them by sending a signal to our immune system to kick into high gear. This triggers inflammation. The body's inflammatory response is its natural defense system. It is there to protect us when we need it, but when the body sees that it is needed regularly it becomes a problem for us in the form of chronic inflammation. You may say, well this is not happening to me because I don't have inflammation. Inflammation does not just mean swollen joints. Here is a list of conditions that are in fact the result of, or linked to inflammation:

IBS

Colitis

autoimmune diseases

allergies

food sensitivities

headaches

brain fog

constipation

acne

recurrent infections

And the list goes on and on. This chronic inflammation can eventually lead to leaky gut and an overall weakened immune system. Leaky gut also leads to inflammation and a weakened immune system. It is a vicious cycle.

Leaky gut is the common terminology for intestinal permeation, meaning that there has been a breakdown of the tight junction of the cells of the intestinal lining. This breakdown allows bacteria, toxins, and undigested food to leak into the bloodstream, which can subsequently trigger an autoimmune response. When the body builds antibodies to the foreign invaders, healthy cells can also take a hit, causing countless other health problems such as poor digestion, fatigue, brain fog, food allergies, autoimmune disorders.

The good news is that damage to the gut can be repaired. I recommend seeing a doctor who is trained in functional medicine if you have any of these ailments or suspect that your gut is in need of repair. They can guide you as to how to eliminate the bad bugs. Once that is done much like turning over a garden you can re-seed by adding good bacteria back into the gut. Again, this should be done under the guidance of an experienced health care professional, such as a naturopath or functional medicine doctor.

Factors that Contribute to Leaky Gut

~Chemicals found in processed foods

~Alcohol and caffeine

~Overuse of antibiotics

~ Eating animal products that have been given antibiotics or hormones

~ Stress

~A diet high in refined sugars contributes to leaky gut. The bad bacteria in your gut love to feed on sugar!

The takeaways:

~ Nix the processed food

~ Choose whole food or foods that don't have a huge list of ingredients, especially if you do not recognize the ingredients as food.

Flush the Tank

So many of the ailments we experience are directly related to our water intake or lack thereof. By simply increasing the amount of water you drink every day, you will help reduce fatigue, feel less hungry, reduce allergy symptoms, headaches, thin mucous, get rid of infections, and aid digestion.

Start your day with at least one glass of water. If you can tolerate two that's even better. For most people it beneficial to drink at least one glass before eating food or drinking coffee as it can help reduce your food cravings. If you don't like the taste of water or if it upsets your stomach try squeezing an orange, lemon or lime to it or for a fresh taste add some cucumber slices and a sprig of mint. You can really add any fruit or spice that makes it taste good to you.

I like to start my day with warm water and lemon or lime. This simple drink can boost the immune system with a shot of vitamin C, aids in digestion and acts as a natural detoxifier. It also flushes the tank so to speak by promoting regular bowel movements.
Another favorite of mine is ginger and turmeric. Both of these roots are used medicinally all over the world. Ginger is packed with vitamins and minerals. It is an antioxidant and has anti-inflammatory properties. Turmeric is a powerful anti-inflammatory. Some studies suggest that it can kill cancer cells and act a pain reliever. Just shave a little of each into warm water (or use the powdered form) with some coconut oil and black pepper and enjoy. This combination is great for inflammation. The point is that in addition to the benefits water has to offer it can be used as a vessel to deliver other nutrients to the body as well.

I'm sure you've heard someone say that you should drink eight glasses of water a day. Presumably 8, eight-ounce glasses. This may be a reasonable goal for most people but again this depends on the individual. Some people require more water than others. Try recording how much water you drink each day for a week. Do this when you are free of illness, injury and are not in excessive weather conditions to gauge what your body requires on average. If you have no interest in drinking or are excessively thirsty it can be a sign that something is amiss within your body so you should see a health care provider to rule out any medical reasons for your thirst.

During times when your body is losing fluids, it is necessary to replenish. It is important to drink before during and after intense or prolonged exercise to keep hydrated. If you are sweating due to exercise or hot/humid weather or illness drinking extra water is vital to preventing dehydration. I always make my kids drink a lot of water the night before a game so they are well hydrated for the event.

Some people have difficulty with waking in the night if they drink water in the evening. Drinking the majority of your water in the morning and afternoon will help to ensure that your sleep is not interrupted with trips to the bathroom.

We want to make sure that our water is pure. Plastic water bottles can contain BPA, which is an endocrine disrupter. When you can, opt for glass or stainless-steel bottles. These are a much better option for you and for the environment too.

Tap water can contain chlorine, fluoride, and lead so it may be worth your while to invest in a water filtration system. There are many types of water filtration systems ranging in size style and cost. Some of the popular types are refillable pitcher filters, faucet systems, carbon water filter and reverse osmosis filters. Do your homework to find a water filter that meets your needs and your budget.

A Tale of Two Crocks: fat-free & lite

For a period of time in my twenties, I almost completely eliminated fat from my diet. Why? Because everything I read told me that fat was bad and carbs were good. It said so on television and in magazines and if it were bad for us then the FDA wouldn't allow it to be advertised as healthy right?

So, there I went eating as much pasta, bagels, and processed fat-free foods as I wanted, including my beloved Snackwells cookies. At this time *fat-free* was all the rage and you could find a fat-free version of almost any food (or pseudo food) as I now call them.

I was lean and looking good, but how I felt was a different story. I was tired all the time and began getting sick a lot. It started with your run-of-the-mill colds and sinus infections, in my twenties but in my thirties, I began getting serious, life-threatening infections, like MRSA, Staph and finally the mother of all infections, CDiff. It was like my immune system had stopped working.

Doctors I saw loaded me up with antibiotics to kill the infections and as each antibiotic stopped working, they upped the ante with a stronger antibiotic. This too wreaked havoc on my gut, destroying all good bacteria along with the bad.

I was diagnosed with a whole host of illnesses and diseases none of which turned out to be accurate. My memory was also suffering. It was like I was in a fog and I was stressed and each and every day was a struggle. Internally I commended myself at the end of each day simply for making it through.

The worst part of all of this was that the fatigue that came with always being sick took a huge toll on me and especially on my parenting abilities. You can have the best intentions but when you feel like shit all the time, it is really hard to see them through. The parent that I wanted to be was not the parent that I was. I was completely exhausted all the time. Then add in the pressure of working a full-time job and caring for kids, husband and elderly parents. My body was in a state of chronic stress and that stress response would also take its toll. It was a recipe for disaster.

In the years following I would learn that my diet, in particular, the fat-free, processed foods were to blame for my original illnesses and then the overuse of antibiotics to treat those ailments destroyed my gut. I would learn that certain vitamins are fat-soluble and the body needs fat to absorb them. I would learn that the brain needs fat to function optimally. None of the articles and advertisements for fat-free and low-fat foods that I read mentioned this. The bottom line is that for years I unwittingly deprived my body of the fat it so desperately needed and replaced it with garbage.

Hopefully, you did not do this to the extreme I did. The good news is, the damage, for the most part, can be undone by simply staying away from these products and eating whole foods. Labeling that boasts 'Fat-free' and 'light' typically means more sugar and more chemicals. Period. End of story. These processed foods have everything bad to offer and nothing good can come of them. Advertising these items as healthy is nothing more than propaganda by big food to sell their products.

Fats

For years we were told by the powers that be that dietary fat translates to body fat and for optimal health low-fat foods were the way to go. This information was false. Fats are important and our bodies need them.

At this point, it seems to be pretty accepted that Mono-unsaturated fats and Poly-unsaturated fats are okay and dare I say offer benefits to our health. It is the other two that we have to worry about, right? You may have heard that you should stay away from saturated fats and trans fats ...and well, I believe this is half true. Saturated fats are not a problem, in fact, we need them. According to Dr. David Perlmutter, "Every cell in your body requires saturated fats; they comprise fifty percent of the cellular membrane. They also contribute to the structure and function of your lungs, heart, bones, liver and immune system."[1]

On the other hand, trans fats are a problem and should be avoided because they are highly processed. To avoid these, eat real food and avoid any packaged or processed food with ingredients that are hydrogenated, such as hydrogenated soybean or vegetable oil. [2]

According to Dr. Mark Hyman, "Naturally

occurring fats in our whole foods aren't the problem; redefined processed fats and oils that are added to our food by the food industry are."[3]

So, the body needs fat but what about our brains? Our brains are comprised of more than seventy percent fat. Then there is the fact that certain fat-soluble vitamins are necessary for brain development and function. So where does that leave our brains without fat? In trouble, that's where. That being said, a great way to eat your fats is along with some veggies. This way you are getting your fat and you are sure to absorb all the nutrients packed inside the veggies. One of my favorites is broccoli and garlic sautéed with coconut oil... delicious!

When choosing fats, it is important to think about the source. If it is animal fat, you need to look not just at the animal, but at what that animal ate because when you eat that animal you are essentially eating whatever they ate. So, if the cow that is now your steak was given antibiotics and hormones you are now consuming those antibiotics and hormones. If a cow is fed corn it makes unhealthy fats, so you are consuming those unhealthy fats. The same way people are meant to eat whole foods, cows are meant to eat grass. When cows graze on grass their bodies convert the grass into healthy fats.

This is why the source of your food matters. Meat should be organic, raised without antibiotics or hormones, free-range, grass-fed and humanely treated. When you eat meat that was sourced this way you receive all the benefits of consuming that animal without anything that you were not asking for. Look for these same criteria when purchasing products that come from the animal such as milk, butter, and eggs.

Good Sources of Fat

Grass-Fed Meat

Wild-caught Fish

Organic Pasture-raised Poultry and eggs

Organic Nuts

Virgin Coconut Oil

Extra Virgin Olive Oil

Avocado

Grass-fed Butter or Ghee (clarified butter)

Bad Sources of Fat

Hydrogenated Oils

Processed and packaged pseudo foods

Carbs

While there are different schools of thought on whether consuming carbohydrates is beneficial, my personal belief is that limiting one's carb intake makes sense for most people. As my teacher, Joshua Rosenthal says, "One person's food is another's poison." Meaning everyone is bio-individual and you need to find what works for you. Remember, balance is important, so too much of any one food will limit your ability to take in nutrients contained in other foods.

Carbohydrates are made up of sugar, starch, and fiber. When you eat carbs your blood sugar rises and the pancreas produces insulin. The human body converts most carbohydrates back into glucose a.k.a sugar. Insulin transports the glucose into the bloodstream where it is absorbed and used for energy. A diet that is low in carbohydrates changes your metabolism so the body burns fat for energy instead of glucose. One way to think of this is that carbs drive insulin and with this, the body is constantly using glucose instead of fat for fuel so the fat hangs around. Usually around your middle;)

Simple vs. Complex Carbs

All carbs are not bad, but keep in mind that not all carbs are created equal. The best source of carbohydrates is those that come from whole foods that are high in fiber such as vegetables, berries, nuts, and seeds. Let's take a quick look.

Simple Carbs Are Sugar

They are burned quickly. Simple carbs cause spikes in blood sugar. Spikes in blood sugar put stress on the body and over time can cause insulin resistance. Some simple carbs occur naturally in foods such as fruits and milk but many that are consumed in the Standard American Diet SAD:(are added to processed foods. Avoiding processed foods including soda, packaged cakes and cookies is important.

Complex Carbs Are Starch and Fiber

These are digested more slowly. They are more nutrient-dense and of course, give you the benefits of fiber. Good sources of complex carbohydrates are green vegetables, sweet and white potatoes, pumpkin, corn (if non-GMO), beans and lentils.

One key point to remember is that during digestion all sugars and starches are turned into sugars. This is something to be mindful of when thinking about how much sugar you are actually consuming. You have to factor in the carbs.

Sugar

I'm going to make this short and sweet ...no pun intended.

Sugar is another hot topic now. There is a great deal of controversy about the effects of sugar, but I believe that in the near future everyone will come to understand the catastrophic effects that too much sugar can have on a person's health.

Hey, I get it that it tastes good. Everyone likes a sweet treat, present company included but unfortunately the more you eat the more you crave. On the flip side, the good news is that the less you eat the less you crave. Once you break the cycle and reduce your sugar intake, you will be amazed at how good you feel. And of course, the source matters.

There are intrinsic or naturally-occurring sugars, which are found in foods like fruits and vegetables. These sugars are digested more slowly so they take longer to enter the bloodstream than free sugars do. This slow and steady release of glucose can help keep blood glucose under control. When consuming this type of sugar, you also have the benefits of the whole food that you are eating including its fiber, vitamins, minerals, antioxidants, protein and calcium. Added sugars or "free sugars," are sugars and sweeteners that are added to foods to make them taste sweeter. These are the sugars that cause rapid spikes in blood sugar.[1]

There are arguments over whether a calorie equals a calorie regardless of the source. The simple answer is that all calories are not equal. Calories that come from added sugars are empty calories. There is nothing positive that these calories have to offer us. While processed foods containing sugar may give you a burst of energy, it will be short-lived and followed by a crash, leaving you hungry again and specifically craving more sugar. It is a vicious cycle.

On the other hand, intrinsic sugars found in fruits and vegetables have benefits. While fruits and vegetables contain sugar, they also come packed with nutrients and fiber we can use to fuel our bodies over the long haul. This type of sugar is absorbed more slowly and therefore it is not turned to fat. So, in a nutshell, what I am suggesting is to always opt for whole fruits and vegetables over any kind of processed food.

Let's look at what some experts say about the effects of sugar on the body. According to Dr. Robert Lustig, a neuroendocrinologist and Professor of Pediatrics in the Division of Endocrinology at the University of California in

San Francisco says, "In the reward center, sugar stimulates the neurotransmitter dopamine, and dopamine drives reward. But dopamine also down-regulates its own receptor (which generates the reward signal). This means the next time around, you're going to need more sugar to generate more dopamine to generate less reward, and so on, until you're consuming a whole lot of sugar, and getting almost nothing for it."[2]

Dr. Mark Hyman, Director of the Cleveland Clinic Center for Functional Medicine, states that sugar is eight times as addictive as cocaine. Dr. Hyman goes on to say, "Being addicted to sugar and flour is not an emotional eating disorder. It's a biological disorder, driven by hormones and neurotransmitters that fuel sugar and carb cravings — leading to uncontrolled overeating." [3]

Not only is sugar considered addictive but it can have a wide range of negative effects on your health. In an article by a doctor of Osteopath and New York Times best-selling author, Dr. Anthony Mercola, he cites seventy-six ways sugar can ruin your health. Among the possible effects that sugar can have on your body he lists the following: interference with the absorption of calcium, magnesium, and protein; a decrease in good cholesterol levels, hyperactivity, and anxiety, difficulty in concentration, drowsiness, and crankiness in children, decreased activity in children, reduction of learning capacity and learning disorders, increased risk of antisocial behavior, a decrease in emotional stability, feeding of cancer cells, increased fasting glucose levels, increased systolic blood pressure, obesity, decreased insulin sensitivity, leading to high insulin levels and eventually diabetes, headaches, including migraines, gastrointestinal tract problems, food allergies, chronic degenerative diseases, atherosclerosis and cardiovascular diseases, autoimmune diseases, such as arthritis, asthma, and multiple sclerosis; toxemia in pregnancy, worsening of symptoms of children with (ADHD) attention deficit hyperactivity disorder, suppression of the immune system, increased risk of contracting infectious diseases, weaker eyesight, premature aging, DNA structure impairment, increased body fluid retention, slowed adrenal gland function, and hormonal imbalance.[4]

I get that it is not realistic for everyone to eliminate sugar from their diet. It is all about balance. Reducing sugar intake, especially free sugars, is a great step to take toward better health and I guarantee you will feel better too. A new World Health Organization guideline recommends adults and children reduce their daily intake of free sugars to less than ten percent of their total calorie intake. They suggest that further reduction to below five-percent or roughly twenty-five grams (or six teaspoons) per day would provide additional health benefits. [5]

Tips to reduce your sugar intake:

1~*Drink more water*. Drinking a glass of water before eating can help reduce the amount of sugar you eat

2~ *When eating sweets opt for sugar from a natural source* rather than food from a box. As far as fruits go, berries and cherries have the lowest glycemic impact and are packed with nutrients. *Berries mixed with some fat can actually slow the release of blood sugar. I love eating blueberries and cashews together as a snack. The sweet and salty mix is delicious.

3~*Eat Sweet Veggies* – like carrots and sweet potatoes because they will naturally help satisfy your sugar cravings

4~*Eliminate processed foods*. They are loaded with sugar not to mention lots of chemicals our bodies don't even recognize.

5~ *Sweeten Creatively*. Using foods and spices that are sweet can help you to cut down on the added sugar you use and, in some cases, even provide you with a health benefit. Try the following to add a sweet flavor to food instead of adding table sugar.

Add Cherries, Dates, Figs, Bananas or another fruit to your baking or to smoothies to get sweetness along with the whole food benefits of nutrients and fiber.

The amazing taste of Pure vanilla extract also serves as an antioxidant, anti-inflammatory, antibacterial agent. [6]

Cinnamon is a natural antioxidant and anti-inflammatory, and it can also help stabilize blood sugar. It has natural antimicrobial, antibiotic, antifungal and antiviral properties and can help to boost the immune system as well. These are just a few of the many health benefits that cinnamon has to offer.[7]

Coconut nectar or coconut sugar contains nutrients and has a lower glycemic index than table sugar so it won't spike blood sugar or make you crash.

Stevia comes from the leaf of the stevia plant. The benefit to using stevia is that it is a whole food with health benefits. It has little to no carbohydrate content and doesn't raise blood sugar.

Good quality dark chocolate contains antioxidants and minerals and is rich in fiber. "The bioactive compounds in cocoa may improve blood flow in the arteries and cause a small but statistically significant decrease in blood pressure." [8]

The sweetness of Monk Fruit comes from naturally occurring antioxidants found in the fruit that have a delicious sweet taste, without the calories of sugar. [9]

Organic raw honey or maple syrup, as these natural sweeteners have antimicrobial properties and are sources of antioxidants, vitamins and minerals and can aid in digestion. [10,11]

Lucuma Powder comes from the lucuma fruit and is considered a superfood because of its medicinal properties. It has a sweet taste but doesn't increase your blood sugar levels. Lucuma powder delivers an abundance of health benefits when added to your favorite food or beverage. "In addition to satisfying your sweet tooth, lucuma is gluten-free and a source of antioxidants, fiber, carbohydrates, vitamins and minerals necessary for bodily functions and of benefit to the immune system." [12]

6~*Quit Soda!* For most things, I say baby steps, but when it comes to soda the sooner you cut it out of your diet the better off you will be. It is poison! Just cutting soda out of your diet without making any other changes will have a positive impact on your body and the way you feel.

Buyer Beware

Some foods that are touted as being organic or healthy contain huge amounts of sugar which may compromise the health benefits of that food. A prime example is yogurt. Some commercial yogurts have more sugar than you should probably consume in a day never mind for one little cup of yogurt. Products like wheat bread can increase blood sugar more than a spoonful of table sugar. Also, beware of "fat-free" or "low-fat" foods. As a general rule of thumb fat-free foods have increased sugar to make up for the lack of taste once the fat is removed. Read labels to ensure that any possible health benefits are not outweighed by tremendous amounts of sugar or chemicals. Try and make a habit of reading the labels and comparing items before putting something in your shopping cart.

To get a good picture of the impact of sugar I highly recommend watching the documentary *FED UP*. And remember...opting for sweet whole foods instead of processed foods that contain added sugars is key.

Protein

There is a huge misconception among the general public when it comes to sources of protein. We have been taught from a very young age that protein comes from meat, period end of story. Well, it's not the end of the story. There are many wonderful plant-based sources of protein as well.

Deciding whether or not to eat meat is a personal choice. It goes back to how some foods that work for some people do not work for others. Some of us want meat in our diet and that is okay. One piece of advice for the carnivores out there ...choose your meat wisely. Meats should be organic, raised without antibiotics or hormones, free-range, grass-fed, grass-finished and humanely treated.

The same way people are meant to eat whole foods, cows are meant to eat grass. When cows graze on grass their bodies convert the grass into healthy fats, but when their diets are altered, they can make unhealthy fats. Grass in their diet is also the way they keep healthy. It's really a no-brainer. Would you like a steak that comes from a healthy cow or a sick cow?

For those opting to be vegetarian or vegan, I have two pieces of advice. First, don't be a junk food vegetarian. These are people who choose not to eat meat but replace it with processed foods instead of other healthy foods. Going down this road will lead to nutrient deficiencies for sure.

Second, be sure you get your protein. While it is possible to get all your necessary nutrients from a plant-based diet, some proteins found in vegetables are not as readily available to the body for absorption as meat proteins. With this in mind, it is important to really do your homework and learn which foods will provide you with the nutrients you need and pay attention to how your body responds to different foods.

Keep an open mind and try new foods. You may be surprised as your taste buds evolve. When I first tried tofu, I thought it was absolutely gross. When my daughter was diagnosed with SIBO her diet was very restricted. Tofu was allowed so I tried it again. I learned that it is all in the way you prepare it. My favorite way is to marinate it in tamari and ginger and then put a light coating of organic, gluten-free flour on it and sauté. I then add it to quinoa and vegetables. It is delicious and my whole family eats it.

A Few Plant Based Protein Sources

Almonds

Broccoli

Spinach

Brown rice

Quinoa

Chickpeas

Black Beans

Kidney Beans

Navy Bean

Pinto Beans

Lentils

Flaxseed

Hemp Seed

Nut butters

Tempeh

Tofu

Gluten

Gluten is a hot topic right now. Some have become gluten-free to be trendy, but for some, it is a necessity. Either way, eliminating or reducing gluten in your diet can definitely serve you well.

Gluten is a group of proteins found in some grains such as wheat, rye, barley, and spelt. Wheat is probably the most popular gluten-containing grain and the one that causes problems for many Americans.

Gluten is used to bind foods together. "Gluten has a sticky attribute that interferes with the breakdown and absorption of nutrients. As you can imagine, poorly digested food leads to a pasty residue in your gut, which alerts the immune system to leap into action, eventually resulting in an assault on the lining of the small intestine."[1] This attack can eventually lead to leaky gut which then puts you at risk for a whole host of other health problems.

Celiac disease is a serious autoimmune disorder that can occur in genetically-predisposed people where the ingestion of gluten leads to damage in the small intestine.[2] While you may not have Celiac disease, it is also possible to have gluten sensitivity. Gluten sensitivity can lead to serious health problems. Among them are

ADHD, anxiety, autoimmune disorders, brain fog, depression, skin irritations, infertility, migraines, neurological disorders such as dementia, Alzheimer's and schizophrenia.

We may not realize the connection between what we eat and how we feel, but I assure you there is a huge connection.

Doing an elimination diet is a good way to determine if you have a gluten sensitivity. In an elimination diet, you eliminate a particular food or food group and gradually introduce it back into your diet. In doing so, you may find some surprising information about how your body reacts to a particular food or food group. In my case, removing gluten from my diet led to a reduction of brain fog and inflammation, and the elimination of headaches, seasonal allergies, and chronic sinusitis. The most impressive result was that my poorly functioning immune system became tremendous. This one took a little more time than the others but I went from being the one who was always sick to hardly even getting a cold.

Removing gluten from your diet will not be easy at first. This is because it is addictive. According to Dr. Perlmutter, "Gluten breaks down in the stomach to become a mix of polypeptides that can cross the blood-brain barrier. Once they gain entry they can bind to the brain's morphine receptor to produce a sensorial high."[3] Dr. William Davis, author of *Wheat Belly*, suggests that when we stop eating grains abruptly it is equivalent to a week of opiate withdrawal.[4] Food manufacturers are well aware of the addictive charms of gluten and they use it to get you hooked on these pseudo foods. In doing so they put money in their pockets at the expense of your health.

You may be wondering why all this is happening when just a few years ago most people didn't even know what gluten was. The answer is simple. The grains we eat now are different from the grains of the past. The food industry has engineered and modified grains which may be less tolerable than those of the past that were free of human tampering. This is one theory about why so many people are finding themselves with Celiac disease or a gluten sensitivity now when this problem seemed to be nonexistent prior to the bio-engineering of foods.

Buyer Beware: According to Dr. Davis, there are very few foods that raise blood sugar higher than gluten. Among the foods that raise blood sugar that high are corn starch, potato starch, tapioca starch, and rice flour.[5] These are the very ingredients you might find in gluten-free processed foods like breads, cakes, and crackers. Just because it says Gluten-free does not mean that it is good for you! The best gluten-free foods are the ones that don't come in a package.

Emotional Eating

As the child of a woman who suffered from mental illness, eating was the only thing I had control over. So, I ate. I ate when I was sad. I ate when I was mad. I ate when I was tired or frustrated. Hell, I ate when I was happy too. And the food I ate was whatever we had in the house. As a very young child, things were good. We had a beautiful garden with lots of fresh vegetables and my diet consisted of home-cooked meals.

My mother, being Italian, cooked wonderful, authentic Italian meals. Unfortunately, as my mother's illness progressed, so did the processed foods we had in the house. Frozen dinners and pre-cooked food in a box or bag became readily available. By the time I was twelve, this became the primary cuisine in our house. My mother stopped making Sunday sauce with braciola and meatballs. She no longer stuffed her own artichokes. She stopped using fresh ingredients from the garden. She stopped making vegetables altogether, except for the occasional canned beets or cold string beans with vinegar and onion flakes. Not very appetizing.

Our main source of food came from a box loaded with salt, sugar, and preservatives. For the most part, my diet consisted of Hot pockets, pizza rolls, and Elios Frozen Pizza. McDonalds and Burger King were big in our house too. I mean it was a win/win, you get dinner and a free drinking glass so there is always a reminder in our cabinet to go back to McDonalds. And of course, go back we did. I mean we had to keep going back to get the complete set of (now vintage) glasses with Ronald, Grimace and the Hamburglar, right? And then there were the free toys which every child wanted and begged their parents to get. Smurfs were my favorite.

Don't get me wrong, there were nights that we opted to go healthy. If we were going for a healthy dinner in my house there was meatloaf, chicken cordon bleu or eggplant parmigiana, all from a box of course. Yes, that's as good as it got. For after school snacks we had a cupboard filled with all the essentials: Doritos, Fritos, Reese's peanut butter cups, and Twix bars. To wash down this wonderful cuisine there was Lipton powdered iced tea, Nestle Quick and Tang (now I am really dating myself). After school, there was that small window of time before my mother got home that

I had peace. It was just me and I was in control...or so I thought. I would start with something cheesy like frozen pizza or pizza rolls, and then move on to the chips, sometimes finishing a whole full-sized bag. After that, I went to the sweet eating which was at least one, but usually two or three candy bars. We always had bananas in the house to go in our morning cereal. Even though Trix, Captain Crunch, and Cocoa Puffs were part of a complete breakfast as the commercial bragged, my dad felt like we needed some fruit in there too. He should have listened to his gut a little more often.

But we were not the only household eating this way. The power of advertising was, and still is, very strong and the majority of American people seem to trust what is advertised on television. After all, we have the FDA and the USDA checking things so there has to be accountability when it comes to food, right? Wrong. The powerful deep pockets of the industry made for a climate of accommodation to these food giants and their purpose at the expense of the American consumer. Media messages would have us believe that Cocoa Puffs and Lucky Charms were 'part of a complete breakfast.' The keyword here being 'part.' They could get away with this statement because technically it could be part of a complete breakfast if that breakfast contained real foods that actually contained nutrients to compensate for the pile of sugar and chemicals in the cereal. And, of course, there was no mention of even the possibility of ill effects from all the sugar and chemicals they were pumping us up with. They made us believe their food was good for us.

This marketing trickery continues today. In my opinion, it contributes to emotional eating. Let's face it, when you are in an emotional state and food is your drug of choice, you are going to be easily swayed. Being constantly bombarded by these persuasive images and messages is like putting someone with a gambling problem in a casino. I believe that many food companies design their marketing around the emotional eater. They are banking on the fact that their campaigns will lead those struggling to make good food choices right to their product in the grocery store. They also rely on the fact that the sugar and chemicals in their product will keep food junkies like me coming back to their product as their 'go-to' food whenever they need a fix.

I fell right into this trap. I was drawn into the commercials of gooey pizza rolls and hot pockets among other things. Eating was the only control I had in my world and I was determined to make it on my terms. I had no idea that what I was putting in my body was slowly killing my immune system, damaging my brain, and would eventually wreak havoc on my whole body.

As an adult, I was breaking down in more ways than one. Thankfully my IIN education saved my life, as I was able to basically detox and get my body back on track. This did not happen overnight and I still struggle. But my struggle is manageable now. I now know what to eat and there are plenty of healthy foods that I enjoy. I am still working on the emotional piece. I share this with you because I have learned that all the education and good intentions in the world will fail if you don't address these two major obstacles. The first is the physiological…why does your body want that food? The second is the psychological aspect of why you turn to food for comfort. What feeling does this food evoke?

Physiological

Our bodies crave different foods for different reasons. In some cases, food cravings exist because of an addiction to that food or group of foods. For example, the more sugar and processed foods we eat, the more we want. Remember, sugar is highly addictive. These foods take us where we want to go mentally, give us a high, but what we don't realize is that the crash that follows is also a direct result of eating the junk.

The more whole plant-based foods you put into your body, the less you will crave junk foods. I believe that a good technique to help you accomplish this is 'crowding out.' [1] This is the process of introducing more good foods so eventually there will be no room for the bad stuff. When I feel a strong craving, I tell myself, "okay you can have it but you have to eat this bowl of greens first." By the time I am finished with the greens, I no longer crave the food I chose for comfort. It is like a switch goes off at some point, and your body recognizes that you will feel like crap after eating crap and you will feel good if you eat good foods.

Psychological

Yesterday, I got some news regarding my daughter's health that was upsetting. This news was not catastrophic and her condition is manageable, so I am grateful for that. Yet with this news came a wave of strong emotions, fear, worry, and relief to some extent that we now know what we are dealing with.

The first chance I got, I found myself in my pantry like an alcoholic with a hidden bottle. I had some junk food in the house that I wouldn't normally buy, but this past Sunday was the Superbowl and I figured I would indulge my guests and my family a little. I should have tossed the leftovers, but instead, I ate them...all of them. Old habits die hard right? Well maybe, but for me, it was more than that. There was a situation (my daughter's health issues) that I had no control over, so I sought control by choosing this food. I reverted back to old behaviors and sought comfort in junk food. Some of these patterns are hard-wired and changing old patterns can be extremely difficult. You may be like me, eating to gain control, or maybe you eat out of boredom or frustration or to fill a need that was not met. You need to figure out your triggers. In order to break the cycle, you have to face your demons.

So, for as much as I have educated myself and made major diet and lifestyle changes my ghosts still occasionally haunt me. I am actively working on these issues but I still have a long way to go. What I know for a fact is that until I have successfully and completely resolved the issues that remain for me, there will be relapses.

Takeaways ~

1-Get support. I recommend working with a professional for this, at least until you can identify what your triggers are. This can be done in an individual or group setting. Emotional eating affects many of us and there is support out there.

2-Find an outlet other than food. Everyone is different in terms of what type of outlet works for them. For me, physical outlets work best, as I need to release my pent-up emotions. Find what works best for you and do it. It may require trying a few different activities to figure it out. Calming activities like painting or yoga may work well for you or you may find your sweet spot doing something where you let it all out like running or kickboxing.

3-Change your relationship with food. Try looking at food in terms of what it can do for you. Think of it as fuel. Are you going to put high-test in your tank so you can go the distance?

4~Don't be sucked in by the advertising that most certainly does not have your best interests at heart.

Navigating the Grocery Store

You want to get the best food possible for your family. There's no question about that. But there is so much coming at you as soon as you enter the grocery store it can be overwhelming. It doesn't have to be though. Here are some simple tips as well as pitfalls to avoid when shopping at the grocery store.

1) **Plan & List.** Plan out your meals for the week and make a list of items to buy. This accomplishes two things. 1-It saves time and prevents you from having to make multiple trips to the store. 2- There are powerful tools of persuasion being used in most grocery stores. Whether you realize it or not you are being bombarded with subtle messages in the form sounds, smells, sales and signs. When you know what you are there for you are more focused and less likely to be swayed by advertising messages within the store.

2) **Don't go food shopping when you are hungry**. You are likely to buy more food and more of the wrong foods.

3) **Shop the Perimeter** The real foods are not in the center of the store. They are around the perimeter. It is here that you will find your produce, meats, fish, poultry and other whole foods. This is where you want to be, my friends. Most of the things in the middle aisles that come in packages are highly processed. If you do opt for items in these aisles try to keep the ingredient list to a minimum. This is what we call 'eating clean.' By doing this you are minimizing the amount of chemicals you put into your body. My general rule is that I will consider it if it has five ingredients or less. Of course, this depends on what the ingredients are.

4) **Create a Colorful Cart**. You should be eating the rainbow so your cart should reflect this. If you see too much beige in your cart it is time to head back to the produce aisle. Remember every fruit and veggie brings something different to the table so eating a diet that is diverse in terms of color and nutritional content can do a body good. Of course, this requires experimentation to see which foods work for you and your family. I like to try a new fruit or vegetable at least every other trip to the grocery store or farmer's market. My kids enjoy this too and it encourages them to try new foods.

5) **Consider the source.** Avoid GMO's. These are foods that are genetically engineered or modified. Look for Non-GMO Project Verified Products to ensure that the food you are buying has not been modified. And yes, there's an app for that. It's called the *Non-GMO Project Shopping Guide*. Fruits and vegetables that are in season are usually an economical choice as well as being fresh and tasty. Also, check out local farmer's markets or consider joining a CSA (Community Supported Agriculture). These are great ways to get fresh, local produce at a reasonable price while supporting your local economy. Buy organic when you can, but realistically organic foods are not always affordable or

accessible for everyone. Conventional produce is better than no produce. The EWG's (Environmental Working Group) Shopper's Guide to Pesticides in Produce provides you with information on which foods are safest to eat in terms of pesticides. And of course, they have an App for that ...EWG's Dirty Dozen, which contain lists they call the Clean fifteen & Dirty dozen. The dirty dozen are foods that you should opt for the organic version when possible because the conventional version contains a significant amount of pesticides and may be genetically modified. The clean fifteen are foods that are okay to buy conventionally. These are handy tools to have on you when you go to the grocery store. Also, remember you have to look at the whole picture. The word organic is not a free pass...check out all the ingredients because the organic label may be only referring to one ingredient.

6) **Labels can lie**. Don't be swayed by labeling that says healthy or natural. This wording is not regulated and can be put on almost anything. Bottom line...if a food or product has to put the word healthy or natural on it, then chances are it's not. Labels can be misleading and many of them are meant to be that way. For example, many products boast the words enriched or fortified. What this means is

that it is processed. It means good stuff was removed during processing and because they put a little back in, they are allowed to call it enriched or fortified. They forgot to mention what the processing does to the food that was once whole. Think about it. Do you really want to buy bread that will last a month because of all the chemicals inside to preserve it? Or do you want fresh bread from a bakery that might only last a couple of days because it doesn't have a ton of chemicals to preserve it? The EWG's Healthy Living App allows you to scan a bar code of a food with your smartphone and get nutritional information on that food.

Road Blocks

The following is a very short chapter, but an important none the less. I would be remiss if I did not mention three things that I call roadblocks. They are thought patterns that do not serve you. These roadblocks are a colossal waste of your time and energy. In fact, they can sabotage any progress you make towards a healthier, more relaxed you. So, do yourself a favor and kick them to the curb!

Anger & Resentment

"I will not be punished by your anger but you will be punished by your anger." ~ Buddha

For a long time, I was angry. As a child, I saw all the families around me and they all looked better than mine. They had moms they could talk to and who talked to them. They had moms that nurtured them and who would kiss a boo-boo instead of screaming at them for getting hurt in the first place. As I got older, I realized that my mother's actions, to some extent, were beyond her control. She was mentally ill. Her severe anxiety had control over every aspect of life. It controlled her thoughts, feelings, actions, and reactions. This extreme anxiety (which we could even call paranoia) was the reason she screamed at me for everything. When I came into a room barefooted, she honestly believed that it would cause me to get very sick and ultimately die of pneumonia. So, she screamed at me, not to be mean, but because the sense of fear she experienced when she saw my bare feet was so intense that she actually felt the need to protect me. (Imagine how much time her sympathetic nervous system was in use). It wasn't until I was an adult that I began to realize that the way my mom treated me was not her fault. Even though I came to have a better understanding of why she did what she did, it didn't make me any less angry. And that anger manifested as stress in my body and mind.

As my mother got older, she developed dementia which intensified her already 'charming' personality. I got even angrier because now I had to care for a woman who never had a nice word to say to me. Again, I know it was not her fault, but I was still angry. This anger manifested itself in many unpleasant ways. I was mentally spent and physically exhausted all the time.

One day I was shopping and I saw this pretty wooden sign. I believe in signs sent from above. This one happened to be an actual physical sign. It said God gave me you. I just stood there staring at it for the longest time. This simple sign was an epiphany of sorts for me. I bought the sign and hung it where I could see it every day to remind me that God put my mother in my life for a reason. Maybe it was because I have the strength to deal with someone like her. Maybe it was to connect me to my father who was the greatest man I've ever known. Maybe it was to show me that we are more than our actions.

Maybe it was to educate me so I know the signs of these illnesses and how to help others. Maybe it was to teach me humility because anyone could end up in her shoes, even me. Or maybe it was to show me how to be grateful. I definitely feel grateful that I don't struggle with these issues myself. I can speculate until the cows come home but the bottom line is that God or the universe or whatever existential being you want to believe in, put this woman in my life for a reason.

So that's it, she was put in my life for a reason and I don't necessarily get to know what that reason is. What I do know is that this is what I got and it is up to me what I do with it. I thought long and hard about it. Was I going to continue to waste my precious energy on being angry? What purpose had my anger served? It certainly didn't change things or make me feel better. What it did do was add more stress to my already very stressful life. So, I decided that I had to find a way to come to terms with it. I decided that moving forward I would do what best serves me, which I knew deep down meant letting go of the anger.

After a lifetime of emotional abuse, turning off the anger toward the source was an enormous challenge. It was not easy to let go of this anger. It was not easy to grasp the notion that from pain comes perspective. After struggling with this for many years I can finally say that I have done it. I let it go. It didn't happen overnight. There was some counseling and some amazing support, but what truly helped me was my faith. Believing in a higher power and greater plan allowed me to sit back and recognize that there is something bigger than me at play here. That being said, there were also several tangible tactics in the form of restorative practices that allowed for a physical and mental release of my anger. Among the greatest tools that worked for me were Qigong, breathwork, meditation and something called Resonance repatterning.

Additionally, physical exercise was an integral part of helping me let go. That physical release is a wonderful outlet for anger without taking it out on other people. All of these practices also helped me to flip my perspective. I now look at this as a pat on the back from God that he knows I am strong enough to handle this. Growing up like this has not defeated me, instead, it has made me stronger. That is the way I look at it now. It gave me perspective on the mental challenges people face. It opened doors for me to study aspects of the brain and mental health. In doing so I have come to help myself and others. This would not have happened if my mother hadn't led me there. So, although difficult, I am no longer angry. I am grateful for my experiences with her because they have made me who I am now. This gratitude and change of perspective have made it possible for me to have empathy for my mother and finally have a positive relationship with her. Granted, with the dementia she doesn't always know who I am, but I know.

Whatever you struggle with, addressing it and moving past anger and resentment is a must. Anger is like an albatross around the neck. It will bring you down physically and emotionally. As I have said before, our energy is precious and if we are devoting any of it to negativity of any kind, we are doing ourselves a disservice.

If you hold any anger or resentment toward yourself or anyone else, find a way to come to terms with it and let it go! For some, this may mean counseling or another form of psychotherapy. For others, restorative practices such as Yoga, Tai Chi, Mediation or Breathwork may be enough. Or, if you're like me, you may need all of those things. The point is to take that first step toward letting go of your anger. It is liberating for both mind and body.

Guilt

If I was at work, I felt guilty for not being with my kids. When I was at home, I felt guilty that I was not at work. I beat myself up for not being the parent I wanted to be, for not being sharper at work, for not being more accommodating to my husband, for everything. My internal self-talk was negative. The underlying message I was feeding myself on a daily basis...you suck, you should be stronger, you should have more energy, you should be able to deal with the pain, you should be better. What I was going through physically was nothing compared to what I was putting myself through mentally as a result of the guilt I felt for being less than perfect.

I have made a lot of changes to better my situation. For the past year, I have been a stay-at-home-mom. During this time, of course, I am caring for my kids, but I have also gone back to school, I am caring for my elderly parents who live with us, and writing this book. With all of this, I still feel guilty that I am not currently bringing in an income.

Guilt is powerful. It is heavy and it can be consuming. It can hinder progress and essentially create a repetitive stress response in the body. Because we have been programmed to do it all, it is easy for women to fall into a pattern of feeling guilty when we are anything less than our version (or someone else's version) of perfect. We can feel guilty for so many things. We all have that little voice in our heads telling us what we should or shouldn't do or say (at least I hope I am not the only one with the little voice:). Some of our inner voices can be very critical and some of us are overrun with the 'should and should not thoughts' such as, "I should be home instead of at work, I should be working instead of at home, I should not eat this, I should not do this, I should have done that, I should not have said that, I should be more ..." And the list goes on.

Externally we apologize to others for our words, actions or lack of actions. Internally we beat ourselves up over what we should have said or done.

These shoulds or should nots can consume us. But what if we just reversed the script? What if our self-talk went something more like this?

> "I am right where I need to be."
>
> "This is delicious and I am going to savor every bite."
>
> "I'm glad I'm doing this."
>
> "Damn right I said that and I'd say it again!"

Can you imagine how different and how liberating that would feel? I've done it and I will tell you it feels good! At first, you may not believe the affirmations you tell yourself, but over time you can become more confident in your choices and know that you can count on your inner wisdom to guide you. It is incredibly empowering to let go of the guilt!

Judgment & Jealousy

There is this mom I would see when picking up my youngest daughter after school. We had met, but I didn't know her well. She looked like perfection with her hair done, beautiful clothes and high heels. She drove a fancy car and carried a little dog around with her. She didn't usually join in conversation with the rest of us moms. We all looked at her like, who the hell does she think she is? We assumed she thought she was better than us. We assumed she was a snob and perhaps we were all a little jealous at how she obviously had plenty of time for herself. The rest of us moms who are burning it at both ends and barely keeping it together resented this type. We thought this woman must have money and everything she wanted but in reality, we knew nothing.

By a random turn of events, one day she and I ended up in the same place at the same time when none of the other moms were around. I was polite and said hello and so did she. Then she began to tell me about the hell that her family had been going through. At first, I thought it odd that she was opening up to me, who was basically a complete stranger to her. Then I realized she was so completely and totally overwhelmed that she saw a friendly face and the floodgates opened. This woman who I thought was spoiled and uppity was anything but that. What I had thought was a bad attitude was not 'attitude' at all. She was wounded and her world was much more complex than any of us could imagine.

She told me of her daughter's life-threatening illness. She told me of how her medical condition had affected her daughter's ability to think and how medications affected her personality making it difficult for her to make friends. She told me of how it breaks her heart to see her daughter on the outside of everything, not knowing how to communicate with the other girls her age. She told me how she and her husband had traveled to find the best medical care for their daughter and how fortunate they felt to have found an amazing surgeon close by in New York. She told me of how seeing her daughter suffers had tested their faith but ultimately it was faith that got them through. Then something crazy happened. She apologized to me. She said she was sorry if she has seemed to be stand-offish but that she is always so focused on her daughter's situation that she hasn't been social.

How crazy is that? This woman who is living every parent's nightmare just apologized to me for not being friendlier to me. I am someone who is insignificant in her life but still, she cared about my feelings. *Wow was I wrong!*

This woman who I had passed judgment on, who I thought was a snob was actually a humble, spiritual, wonderful human being who was hurting on a level I could not even grasp. I was floored! I thought I was a good judge of character but I was so far off the mark it was ridiculous. I walked away thankful for this conversation and realizing two things. One, that God puts people in your path for a reason. I was feeling overwhelmed and down. I believe this happened to help me gain perspective and realize the gifts in my life. Two, no matter what things look like, don't judge. I know that is easy to say but hard to do. The fact is we simply don't know people's real story. More often than not we have no clue what life experiences they have had or even what they may currently be going through. It is human nature to assess people and make a judgment, but I urge you to remember this woman and think twice before doing so without the facts.

Judgment and jealousy are a waste of our precious energy.

Removing Road Blocks

There are a few practices that I believe will help you remove any roadblocks. Each of them involves putting ourselves out there a little bit and a letting go. To move forward we must let go of repetitive patterns that do not serve us and try to change the dance. It is a bold move to let go of the security that comes with keeping the status quo.

Lose the Clutter

Get rid of clutter. This means clutter in your mind and clutter in your physical space. When you eliminate clutter, you eliminate one huge source of stress.

Did you ever hear the saying, 'Don't sweat the small stuff?' Well, this really applies here. We need to get rid of the things that are clogging up our heads especially those negative thoughts or thoughts about things you have no control over. There is a saying in qigong... "Where the mind goes the qi flows." This means when you constantly think about something, your precious energy is being spent on those thoughts.

When you think of it this way, wouldn't you rather your energy and resources go toward something positive, something that will benefit you? In order to accomplish this, you can engage in any restorative practice, such as Qigong or Tai Chi, Meditation, breathwork, exercise, guided imagery or yoga. Any creative outlet will help you relax and focus on the positive.

The other thing is to simply let it go. Breathe in, breathe out and let go of the feelings that don't serve you. Negative or self-limiting thoughts do not serve your best interest. As hard as it may be to let go of anger and resentment you must find a way or they will become toxic. You can try this very simple exercise of utilizing self-talk. When you start to think a negative thought, simply replace it with a positive one. This will take some practice.

For example, replace a thought like, "Oh shit it's freezing outside. I hate the cold," with "One more cold day under our belts means one day closer to spring and warm weather." This will divert your anger and help you become calmer and more relaxed, returning you to the parasympathetic nervous system where you can definitely reap the benefit.

Now the physical space. Along with clearing your head, clearing your physical space can go a long way toward peace of mind. Sometimes it's hard to part with our 'stuff,' but getting rid of things that you have no use for can be a great start. Try cleaning out a closet, reorganizing your office, or even just cleaning out a drawer. Not only will you breathe a sigh of relief when it is done (hopefully a belly breath) but it will be one less thing to worry about. This can free up some much-needed mental space too!

Accolades

"Two kinds of gratitude: The sudden kind we feel for what we take; the larger kind we feel for what we give." ~ Edwin Arlington Robinson

How do you feel when you receive a compliment? While I do subscribe to the mantra, 'don't worry about what others think of you,' I have to admit when someone compliments me it feels pretty damn good. Affirmations empower us. They raise us up a little bit and can make a big difference for someone who is struggling or even just having a bad day.

Compliments are a form of gratitude. I was talking with my mother's speech therapist and out of nowhere she said, "You look really fit, you must take good care of yourself." I thought it odd as we were discussing my mother's care plan and this was a random comment, but then she said something else that has stuck with me. She said, "A friend once told me if you are thinking something nice about someone, say it out loud. It doesn't take any big effort on your part and chances are it will make them feel really good."

It doesn't get any simpler than that, but how true that is. When you compliment someone, it shows an appreciation for some aspect of who they are, or maybe for them in general and this is incredibly powerful.

A few words of praise can truly lift someone up. The funny thing about this is that it is twofold because not only will you make the other person feel great, you will feel great you when you go out of your way to compliment someone. This woman was a genius. She was absolutely right. It doesn't take much on our part to compliment someone but just wait until you see the reward you get. Call it karma, call it what you will…it works!

Let me give you a couple of examples. I recently ran into an old friend who I hadn't seen in a while so we chatted but I could sense she was not herself. I mentioned to her how great her skin looked. It was not a big thing, but to her it was. Whatever was going on for her that day was bringing her down. She didn't go into it but you could feel her mood. That little compliment brought a big smile to her face. "Really?" she asked. "Absolutely," I said. "It is like you are glowing." At that point, her whole effect changed. She definitely left our little conversation in a better place than she was when it started. It took nothing for me to make this comment, but to her, it was something special.

One day at a physical therapy session I had a conversation with another patient. I don't remember too much about the conversation other than talking about our injuries and our kids. I made him laugh a couple of times. The conversation was nothing earth-shattering. I was getting ready to leave, so I said goodbye and told him it was nice to meet him. He said the same, but as I was about to walk away, he said, "I really enjoyed talking to you." I ran into him again at the appointment desk and he reiterated his sentiment with a lot of enthusiasm. He said, " Take care of yourself and again I really enjoyed talking with you." I cannot even tell you how good this made me feel. He could not have made me feel better if he said I was beautiful or brilliant.

I think as moms we often feel like we are not heard so having someone take the time to engage in a conversation with me was nice, but then to tell me how much he enjoyed talking to me, well that was the bomb. The fact that this happened more than a year ago and I am now writing about it tells you what an impact it had on me. For the life of me, I can't remember his name or what we talked about but I can remember how great I felt after that compliment. It made me feel so good about myself, not just in that moment but for the rest of the day and probably for a couple of days after. Why? Because when someone tells you they value any aspect of you it makes you feel good.

The three experiences I just described were simple little interactions with people I hardly knew, but as you can see, they moved me. I began trying to make a point of complimenting my loved ones and people I hardly knew. It really took no effort because I was simply saying out loud what I was thinking anyway.

I can honestly say that as nice as it is to receive a compliment, giving a compliment is actually more gratifying. Letting people know you appreciate them will enhance your mood and maybe even make you a little more grateful for who you are and who you connect with. The same holds true with a random act of kindness. When we do something nice for someone without expecting anything in return it gives us a feeling of connection to others. This connection helps us to feel like we are part of something bigger than ourselves. Give it a try.

Gratitude

"At times, our own light goes out and is rekindled by a spark from another person. Each of us has cause to think with deep gratitude of those who have lighted the flame within us."

– Albert Schweitzer

Gratitude is a form of self-love. Gratitude can take many forms. Appreciating those who make a difference in our lives seems like a given, but in the business of our lives, this simple practice can be lost. Whether it is an "I love you" or "you make me laugh" or "you played a great game today" or any other form of affirmation, it has great value. When we practice recognizing the people and good things in our lives, and even the good that has come out of a bad situation we are really feeding our souls.

We kind of expect our kids to take us for granted the same way we took out parents for granted. It's almost like a rite of passage. I figure maybe somewhere in their thirties they will appreciate some aspect of our existence. So that being said, I was blessed with an exception to this rule. Her name is Isabella. She is the feisty one and can be quite sassy at times. For the most part, she is like any other kid doing her own thing, except that she is not.

From a very young age, without being asked or taught, she has shown gratitude for the people in her life, for experiences she has had, and for me in particular. She thanks me for things I don't expect a thank you for and would never get one from anyone else. She thanks me for all the things that moms just do, like cooking her something she likes, doing her laundry, driving her somewhere, rubbing her back when she is sick or cleaning up after her. It is not just the thank you though, it is the way she says it and how she looks at me and hugs me when she says it.

I can feel her love and appreciation. So, I can honestly say that a four-year-old taught me gratitude. She taught me to appreciate and she has reinforced this lesson over and over again. I will always be grateful to her, and for her.

Recently, we took our oldest son Jack to college. I have always been grateful for him, but never have I felt this more than I do right now. I know I have not lost my son, yet there is still a sense of loss. He is on his own now, and while he still needs me in some respect it is profoundly different. I am not spending time with him every day, or tending to his every need. This was a part of my purpose and it is hard to lose that piece of me. He now resides in a different state and I miss him terribly. It is probably the strangest feeling I have ever had. On one hand, I am heartbroken that I don't get to be with him every day, but at the same time, I am incredibly proud of his many accomplishments and the young man that he has become. While always being very driven and going after what he wants, he has been able to maintain the kindness and compassion he has always shown for others. I am grateful that for all the changes in his life he is still the same witty old soul he has always been. I am also excited for him to start his own life's journey and for all his new experiences, and am grateful for the opportunities that await him. But above all, I am just so damn grateful that I have been blessed to have him in my life and I believe it is this gratitude that gets me through.

I am grateful for my daughter, Jordyn's passion and ability to give her all to whatever she does. Whether it is hockey, lacrosse, school work or a friendly game of cards with her grandfather, she is all in. I am especially grateful for her resilience. She has faced more challenges than any child should have to. She is like Rocky Balboa though. Each time she gets knocked down she just keeps getting back up. She has worked so hard when I think many would have thrown in the towel. She has kept her drive, her spirit and most importantly her sense of humor through it all. I am beyond grateful for this.

When we experience a loss, it gives us perspective on what we had. I really felt this when my dad died. I was always grateful for him but how often I shared my feelings with him did not reflect the magnitude of how I felt. As they say, hindsight is 20/20, but if I could go back, I would leave no doubt in his mind. He would not just have to assume it. He would hear from me regularly about what an incredible gift he is in my life. Maybe thinking about what life would be like without the people in our life is a good way to gain more appreciation for them.

I'm not suggesting that anyone doesn't appreciate their family and friends, but let's face it, life is busy and we all take what we have for granted to a certain extent. Taking a minute to recognize the people in your life and what they bring to your life is a good way to gain a perspective which will lead you to gratitude. And letting them know you appreciate them can build connections and improve relationships.

On any given day there is a lot we can complain about. But let's try to change the dance! When you feel frustrated or unappreciated, stop and take a look around you. Notice all the good there is. Respond to someone in a new and different way. Sometimes responding in a way that is unexpected can change the whole dynamic of a situation. This is especially true when we are in a repetitive pattern that is not serving us. For example, let's say your mother-in-law always comments on what you can do better when it comes to your home or children.

You work very hard to be the best parent you can be and make a nice home for your family, so this is very insulting to you. Your normal reaction might be to tell her where to go, or worse to say nothing and let the anger fester internally. Instead, try saying something like, "I will take that under advisement," or just throwing a compliment her way. I know it sounds strange but this type of unexpected response can change the entire direction of a conversation. She was not expecting a compliment so she is thrown off guard and in turn, has to alter her response to fit your new and unusual response.

"Studies show we can deliberately cultivate gratitude, and can increase our well-being and happiness by doing so. In addition, gratefulness—and especially expression of it to others—is associated with increased energy, optimism, and empathy." [1]

It can be difficult to feel gratitude when you feel like life is not going the way you wanted it to. It may take some time before you can appreciate a situation that is less than optimal, but if you try to pull something positive despite the negative eventually there will be a paradigm shift. Your way of thinking can evolve.

For example, let's consider another scenario. Say you don't feel appreciated or supported by your husband. I think it's fair to say that a lot of women can relate to this feeling. Your thoughts and feelings toward him may start to take on negativity. But what if, instead of focusing on what he doesn't give you, at least once a day you tell yourself something positive that he brings to the table. Dig deep, find something, anything! Even if it is just that he takes out the garbage, celebrate it in your mind as if that is the most wonderful thing he could do. Even if you have to make it funny…who needs to be wined and dined… I never have to worry about the garbage going out on Tuesdays. This way you create positive thoughts, you are cultivating gratitude, and the situation may even give you a good laugh. We know how important that is.

Conclusion

While this is a self-help book, one of the biggest take-aways is that everything we do as parents is modeling for our children. When it comes to our daughters.... How we care for ourselves or don't care for ourselves is what they are learning to be the norm. If they see us running ourselves ragged and not taking care of our bodies and minds, we are telling them this is acceptable. They will view this way of life as what is expected of a wife and mother. The same holds true for our sons. If they see their mother as the sacrificial lamb, then this is how they will treat their wife or partner. They will expect the world from their female (or male) counterpart and bring little to the table. This will set the stage for a repetitive pattern. As I am sure you do, I want better for my children.

I want them to know that they have choices and they have a voice. I want them to take the time to appreciate the simple things in life. I want them to give of themselves to care for others, but I also want them to nourish themselves. I want them to be in touch with who they are because that is the only way to truly connect with others. I want them to live life to the fullest whatever that means for them. I want them to speak their truth and not try to fit who they are into someone else's view of who they should be. I want them to feel a sense of peace. I want them to have the tools to take care of their own physical and mental health. When there is internal conflict and storms arise, as they will, I want them to be able to go inward and be still. I want them to know there are many things in life that are beyond our control and letting go and trusting them to God or the universe is sometimes necessary. I want them to know there is a reason for all our experiences. Most importantly, I want them to feel loved for being exactly who they are.

The way we can teach this to our children is to live this way, ourselves. In doing so we care for our precious selves as we pave the way for the next generation to do the same.

I hope you have enjoyed reading this book and have gotten some useful information to take with you. I hope that this has book has helped you to know you are not alone on your journey. Most of all, I hope it has helped you get to a place where you will begin nourishing yourself because you deserve it.

REFERENCES

CHAPTER 2: ADDRESS THE MEDICAL

Clean Up the Endocrine

[1.] Kresser, Chris. "Five Thyroid Patterns That Won't Show Up on Standard Lab Tests." *Kresser Institute*, Kresserinstitute.com, 4 May 2018, kresserinstitute.com/why-your-normal-thyroid-lab-results-may-not-be-normal/.

[2.] Levy, Jillian. "6 Steps to Get Your Cortisol Levels Under Control & Turn Down the Stress." *Dr. Axe*, 14 June 2018, draxe.com/cortisol-levels/.

[3.] Kresser, Chris. "Adrenal Fatigue or HPA Axis Dysregulation?" *Kresser Institute*, Kresserinstitute.com, 2 May 2018, kresserinstitute.com/adrenal-fatigue-hpa-axis-dysregulation/.

Brain Fog

[1 & 2.] Perlmutter, David. *Grain Brain*. Yellow Kite, 2015.

CHAPTER 3: SELF ACCEPTANCE

Speak Your Truth

[1.] Gmitter, Aria. "25 Powerfully Inspirational Quotes Prove That Vulnerability Makes Us Stronger." *YourTango*, 26 Jan. 2018, www.yourtango.com/2016297537/25-powerful-inspirational-quotes-prove-vulnerability-makes-us-stronger?utm_source=contentstudio.io&utm_medium=referral.

[2.] John Mayer. "Say." *Say*, John Mayer, Steve Jordan, The Village, LA, California, 20 Nov. 2007.

Set the Stage

Thrive

[1] Weaver, Libby. *Rushing Woman's Syndrome: How to Stay Healthy with a Never-Ending to-Do List*. Hay House Pub, 2017.

CHAPTER 4: NOURISHING YOU

Breathe

[1] Palma, Zandra. "What Is Breathwork and Does It Work? A Doctor Explains the Science." *Parsley Health*, 9 Apr. 2019, www.parsleyhealth.com/blog/breathwork-does-it-work/.

[2] Weil, Andrew. "The Art and Science of Breathing - Dr. Weil." *DrWeil.com*, 17 Oct. 2017, www.drweil.com/health-wellness/balanced-living/meditation-inspiration/the-art-and-science-of-breathing

Cultivate Good Smells

[1] Psychology Today. "The Hidden Force of Fragrance." *Psychology Today*, Sussex Publishers, 1 Nov. 2007, www.psychologytoday.com/us/articles/200711/the-hidden-force-fragrance.

[2] "The Smell Report." *The Smell Report - Emotion.*, www.sirc.org/publik/smell_emotion.html.

[3] "Exploring Aromatherapy." *NAHA*, naha.org/explore-aromatherapy/about-aromatherapy/what-is-aromatherapy.

[4] Snyder, Mariza. *Smart Mom's Guide to Essential Oils: Natural Solutions for a Healthy Family, Toxin-Free Home and Happier You*. Ulysses Press, 2017.

[5] Axe, Josh. "Lemongrass Essential Oil Uses & Benefits, for Skin, Hair & More." *Dr. Axe*, 28 Nov. 2018, draxe.com/lemongrass-essential-oil/.

Exercise

[1] Harvard Health Publishing. "Exercising to Relax." *Harvard Health*, www.health.harvard.edu/staying-healthy/exercising-to-relax.

[2] Kahn, Joel. "Why Sweating Is The Best Way To Get Rid Of Toxins." *Mindbodygreen*, Mindbodygreen, 13 July 2015,

Thrive

www.mindbodygreen.com/0-15166/why-sweating-is-the-best-way-to-get-rid-of-toxins.html.

Find Your Tribe

1. Buettner, Dan. *The Blue Zones: 9 Lessons for Living Longer from the People Who've Lived the Longest*. National Geographic, 2012.

Laugh

1. "Laughter Therapy History: Who, What, When." *Laughter Online University*, 8 Dec. 2018, www.laughteronlineuniversity.com/western-history-laughter-therapy/.

2. American Physiological Society. "Laughter Remains Good Medicine." *ScienceDaily*, ScienceDaily, 17 Apr. 2009, www.sciencedaily.com/releases/2009/04/090417084115.htm.

3. "6 Reasons Why Laughter Is the Best Medicine." *The Chopra Center*, 24 Feb. 2017, www.chopra.com/articles/6-reasons-why-laughter-is-the-best-medicine#sm.00009q0fhzrn4em6qv115j3r7fadp.

Say Yes to the O!

1. "Women's Sexual Health: Talking about Your Sexual Needs." *Mayo Clinic*, Mayo Foundation for Medical Education and Research, 18 Apr. 2017, www.mayoclinic.org/healthy-lifestyle/sexual-health/in-depth/womens-sexual-health/art-20047771.

2. Brighton, Jolene. "Why an Afternoon Delight Is Good for Women's Health." *Dr. Jolene Brighten*, 28 Feb. 2019, drbrighten.com/why-orgasms-are-good-for-women-how-to-improve-your-libido/.

CHAPTER 5: NUTRITION

Food for Pleasure & Power

1. Food Matters. "What's Really In A Big Mac?" *FOOD MATTERS®*, Food Matters, 21 Oct. 2018, www.foodmatters.com/article/whats-really-in-a-big-mac.

Grandma's Rolling

1. It, Just Label. "Just Label It." *Just Label It*, www.justlabelit.org/.

2. https://www.federalregister.gov/documents/2018/12/21/2018-27283/national-bioengineered-food-disclosure-standard

3. "Choose MyPlate." *Choose MyPlate*, www.choosemyplate.gov/.

4. Nestle, Marion. *Food Politics*. University of California Press, 2007.

5. Simon, Michele. *Appetite for Profit: How the Food Industry Undermines Our Health and How to Fight Back*. Nation Books, 2006.

Flush the Tank

1. "Water: How Much Should You Drink Every Day?" *Mayo Clinic*, Mayo Foundation for Medical Education and Research, 6 Sept. 2017, www.mayoclinic.org/healthy-lifestyle/nutrition-and-healthy-eating/in-depth/water/art-20044256.

2. Rosenthal, Joshua. *Integrative Nutrition: Feed Your Hunger for Health & Happiness*. Institute for Integrative Nutrition, 2014.

Fats

1. Perlmutter, David. *Grain Brain*. Yellow Kite, 2015.

2. Hyman, Mark. *Food: What the Heck Should I Eat?* Little, Brown and Company, 2018.

Sugar

1. "The Science behind the Sweetness in Our Diets." *World Health Organization*, World Health Organization, 30 Oct. 2014, www.who.int/bulletin/volumes/92/11/14-031114/en/.

2. Lustig, Robert H. "The Sugar-Addiction Taboo." *The Atlantic*, Atlantic Media Company, 30 May 2018, www.theatlantic.com/health/archive/2014/01/the-sugar-addiction-taboo/282699/.

3. "How to Curb Cravings for Good." *Dr. Mark Hyman*, 8 Jan. 2019, drhyman.com/blog/2019/01/07/how-to-curb-cravings-for-good/.

4. "76 Scary Things That Can Happen inside Your Body Every Time You Put Sugar in Your Mouth." *Mercola.com*, articles.mercola.com/sugar-addiction.aspx.

5. "WHO Calls on Countries to Reduce Sugars Intake among Adults and Children." *World Health Organization*, World Health Organization, 17 May 2016, www.who.int/mediacentre/news/releases/2015/sugar-guideline/en/.

6. Edwards, Rebekah. "The #1 Anti-Inflammatory Extract for Your Medicine Cabinet (Make It Easily at Home)." *Dr. Axe*, 23 Oct. 2016, draxe.com/vanilla-extract/.

7. Axe, Josh. "13 Major Cinnamon Benefits Explain Why It's the World's No. 1 Spice." *Healthy Diet Portal*, 25 Feb. 2019, healthydietportal.com/13-major-cinnamon-benefits-explain-why-its-the-worlds-no-1-spice/.

8. Gunnars, Kris. "7 Proven Health Benefits of Dark Chocolate." *Healthline*, Healthline Media, www.healthline.com/nutrition/7-health-benefits-dark-chocolate.

9. "WHAT IS MONK FRUIT?" *Monkfruit.org*, Monkfruit.org, 2 July 2015, monkfruit.org/what-is-monk-fruit-2/.

10. "What Are the Benefits of Raw Honey?" *Mercola.com*, foodfacts.mercola.com/raw-honey.html.

11. "Positive and Negative Effects of Honey on the Body." *LIVESTRONG.COM*, Leaf Group, www.livestrong.com/article/440371-positive-and-negative-effects-of-honey-on-the-body/.

12. "Benefits of Lucuma Powder." *LIVESTRONG.COM*, Leaf Group, www.livestrong.com/article/479259-benefits-of-lucuma.

Gluten

1 & 3. Perlmutter, David. *Grain Brain*. Yellow Kite, 2015.

[2] "What Is Celiac Disease?" *Celiac Disease Foundation*, celiac.org/celiac-disease/understanding-celiac-disease-2/what-is-celiac-disease/#Fvgg1uCrpo14X4jA.99.

[4 & 5] Davis, William. *Wheat Belly: Lose the Wheat, Lose the Weight, and Find Your Path Back to Health*. Rodale Books, 2019.

Emotional Eating

[1] Rosenthal, Joshua. *Integrative Nutrition: Feed Your Hunger for Health & Happiness*. Institute for Integrative Nutrition, 2014.

Navigating the Grocery Store

[1] "Verified Products." *The NonGMO Project*, livingnongmo.org/find/products/.

[2] "EWG." *EWG*, www.ewg.org/.

CHAPTER 6: STRESS

Stress & Your Body

[1] "How Chronic Stress Creates Hormonal Havoc." *Dr. Mark Hyman*, 8 Jan. 2015, drhyman.com/blog/2014/11/25/chronic-stress-creates-hormonal-havoc/.

[2] Harvard Health Publishing. "Relaxation Techniques: Breath Control Helps Quell Errant Stress Response." *Harvard Health*, www.health.harvard.edu/mind-and-mood/relaxation-techniques-breath-control-helps-quell-errant-stress-response.

[3] "Dr Libby: How Stress Affects Your Food Choices." *Stuff*, www.stuff.co.nz/life-style/well-good/teach-me/82630883/Dr-Libby-How-stress-affects-your-food-choices.

Stressbusters

[1] "Laughter Therapy History: Who, What, When." *Laughter Online University*, 8 Dec. 2018, www.laughteronlineuniversity.com/western-history-laughter-therapy/.

Harvard Health Publishing. "Relaxation Techniques: Breath Control Helps Quell Errant Stress Response." *Harvard Health*, www.health.harvard.edu/mind-and-mood/relaxation-techniques-breath-control-helps-quell-errant-stress-response.

CHAPTER 8: REMOVING ROADBLOCKS

Gratitude

1. "Gratitude." *Psychology Today*, Sussex Publishers, www.psychologytoday.com/basics/gratitude.

ABOUT THE AUTHOR

Dina Vecchione Milne is a Health Coach, social worker, and author. She received her Health coaching training from the Institute for Integrative Nutrition. As the founder of Intrinsic Synergy, LLC, she's passionate about helping women who are trying to keep up with the overwhelming demands put upon them in modern society. Dina's goal is to inspire women to improve their physical and emotional health by practicing self-care. Clients describe her as "compassionate" "inspiring" and "motivating." For more information or to stay in the know, visit www.intrinsicsynergy.com

This book was inspired by my experience at the Institute for Integrative Nutrition® (IIN), where I received my training in holistic wellness and health coaching. IIN offers a truly comprehensive Health Coach Training Program that invites students to deeply explore the things that are most nourishing to them. From the physical aspects of nutrition and eating wholesome foods that work best for each individual person, to the concept of Primary Food – the idea that everything in life, including our spirituality, career, relationships, and fitness contributes to our inner and outer health – IIN helped me reach optimal health and balance. This inner journey unleashed the passion that compels me to share what I've learned and inspire others. Beyond personal health, IIN offers training in health coaching, as well as business and marketing. Students who choose to pursue this field professionally complete the program equipped with the communication skills and branding knowledge they need to create a fulfilling career encouraging and supporting others in reaching their own health goals. From renowned wellness experts as Visiting Teachers to the convenience of their online learning platform, this school has changed my life, and I believe it will do the same for you. I invite you to learn more about the Institute for Integrative Nutrition and explore how the Health Coach Training Program can help you transform your life. Feel free to contact me to hear more about my personal experience at www.intrinsicsynergy.com/integrativenutrition or call (844) 315-8546 to learn more.

Made in the USA
Middletown, DE
13 August 2020

14728767R00135